BEYOND DIGESTION

BEYOND
DIGESTION

*How GUT Health Connects
to Your Mind, Body, and Soul*

DR. LAURA M. BROWN, ND

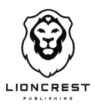

LIONCREST

PUBLISHING

MEDICAL DISCLAIMER: The information contained in this book is intended for educational purposes only. Individuals should always see their healthcare provider before administering any suggestions made in this book. Any application of material set forth in the following pages is at the reader's discretion and sole responsibility.

BEYOND DIGESTION
How GUT Health Connects to Your Mind, Body, and Soul

ISBN   978-1-5445-1847-3 *Hardcover*
          978-1-5445-1846-6 *Paperback*
          978-1-5445-1845-9 *Ebook*

For those who need help digesting food and the world around them.

CONTENTS

INTRODUCTION

Your gut contains ten times as many microbes as your whole body contains human cells. That means 99 percent of the genes in your body come from microbes. In voting terms, that is a ton of influence on your life. Newsflash! If you can influence the microbes, you can influence your entire being. In this book, you will meet plenty of folks who found that when they reset their gut, they reset their life.

Folks like Jeanie, who lost 25 pounds in six months and slowed her progression of multiple sclerosis. Paul, who solved his diarrhea. Samantha, who resolved her sinus and eye issues. Nancy, who eliminated her recurring body-wide hives. Stephanie, who lost 20 pounds and reversed fatty liver disease in four months. Sam, who figured out his lifelong constipation, thinks more clearly, and no longer walks with a cane. Sonja, who reclaimed her energy. Maxwell who solved his tremors and feels confident to go out on a date. And Amanda, who is liberated to use her vacation days for vacation instead of sick days!

This is an in-depth guide for *your* health.

It's about digestion, food, and the world around you.

How does gut health relate to the health of the rest of your body, mind, and soul?

Two thousand four hundred fifty years ago, Hippocrates said, "It all begins in the gut." I think he was smarter than even he knew. Has the human condition changed at all since then?

The onset of digestive and gastrointestinal issues often begins in times of grief, abuse, or other major negative life events. As Dr. Samuel Gee says, "What the patient takes beyond his ability to digest does him harm." I found that quote after years of encapsulating what I do by saying, "I help people better digest their food and the world around them."

I'm going to show you why the health of your digestive tract is critical to your enjoyment of life. The state of the gut is the root of many chronic health issues. Even your mood can be a reflection of or reaction to what is going on in your gut.

The promise of the book is to *help you appreciate that your mood and overall health could be determined by your gastrointestinal health*. It could be that treating symptoms doesn't get to the heart of the matter. It is time to stop putting on Band-Aids and take a long look under the hood. Society spends billions treating chronic disease in North America, and still people are not well.

According to the American Association of Anxiety and Depression:

Seventy percent of people with irritable bowel syndrome (IBS) are not receiving treatment.

- Of the 30 percent who do seek treatment, 50–90 percent suffer from anxiety or depression.[1]
- Forty million adults between 18 and 54 years of age seek help for anxiety.[2] That's almost 20 percent of the population.

What if one of those people is you?

That's the real picture.

Let's get real.

As Victor E. Frankl once said, *"When we are no longer able to change a situation, we are challenged to change ourselves."*

It's up to you to decide if you are ready to change yourself.

Are you?

I'm talking about small incremental changes as well as bigger commitments to better your health.

It's about evolution, not revolution.

Change can be difficult.

Most people don't like change.

---

1   https://adaa.org/about-adaa/press-room/facts-statistics, accessed September 3, 2019.

2   https://adaa.org/about-adaa/press-room/facts-statistics, accessed September 3, 2019.

But what if you don't like where you are either?

"You can't go back and change the beginning, but you can start where you are and change the ending."

—C. S. LEWIS

Healing is a step-by-step process, like peeling the layers of an onion. In order to heal, you have to go one layer at a time. It might even make you cry! It involves addressing the physical, emotional, cognitive, and spiritual levels.

There is a lot packed into this read. You may choose to read it in sections. You may even choose to read it a number of times. That's because at different phases in your journey, you are naturally ready to learn and work on different areas. Peeling the onion takes time and effort.

My goal is to help you recognize patterns, remove obstacles, and stimulate your body's natural mechanisms to repair damage and rebuild health.

You can only make decisions based on what you know. As you learn new information, you integrate it with your prior knowledge and apply it to your current experience. It's an evolutionary process. We learn as individuals, but we also learn as a collective generation. We have advanced in what we know about digestion, but we have also wandered from a lifestyle that supports the common blueprint of our being.

We know more intellectually, but we sadly lack the wisdom to care for our bodies.

It seems the more we fill our brains with knowledge, the further we get from living how our bodies love us to live. Take diet, for example. We know way more about the effects of fats and carbohydrates and proteins than we ever have. But do we eat better? Or do we try to get away with more, like teens pushing the limits of a curfew? There are universal guidelines we keep trying to outsmart, and the result is usually a swift kick in the pants.

To protect their privacy, I have changed names and identifiers of patients sharing their stories. The sad thing is, their conditions are not uncommon, so it could be anyone struggling with digestive issues, emotional regulation, or a chronic disease.

MEET JAMIE

Jamie, 35, is a married teacher and mother of two. When she comes to see me, she is 25 pounds overweight and struggling with IBS. Her recent lab results show progression in autoimmune disease. She has frequent headaches and feels self-conscious about the eczema patches on her face and neck. She was diagnosed with hypothyroidism at age 15 and has been on levothyroxine since. She is also on oral birth control. When she was 21, she slipped and fell and injured her neck. Head and neck tension are frequent. Work is stressful, and whenever the workload increases, her bowels go from slow to moving three to five times a day. She gets a pain in her gut after arguing with her husband. Sometimes so bad she has to take the next day off work.

Anxiety rears its head every day, especially in the afternoon. Sometimes it rises again at bedtime and makes it hard for her to fall asleep. Coffee is her friend, and she *loves* anything sweet.

She feels guilty when she gives in and then tries to make up for it by eating something healthy but more often ends up skipping the next meal entirely.

She feels self-conscious about the skin rashes, although she knows this is more about her vanity than anything else. She's overwhelmed with stress from balancing work and home and struggles to uphold standards for her relationships. She needs a better way than food to deal with stress.

Even on an average day, Jamie is uncomfortable and embarrassed because of her gas and urgency.

Her family has a lakeside cottage, and she's looking forward to a vacation there. She'd like to be able to go canoeing and waterskiing without worrying about having to use the bathroom.

With at least 70 percent of the immune system residing in the gut, there is little wonder that her immune system is weak; it is intricately linked to sugar consumption and gut health.

Ingestion of contaminated water while at the cottage can also put Jamie at risk for bacterial or protozoa infection, which can not only contribute to IBS but also generate off-gas toxins that leak out of the gut and can wind up in the brain.

Jamie doesn't realize that the medications she is on affect the microbiome. At the same time, if she doesn't manage her thyroid well, low levels of thyroid hormone can affect the gut motility and make constipation worse. And as for birth control, one child from each marriage is enough, thank you very much. Coffee can help with constipation; however, too much can be like a cup of stress. Hypothyroidism and autoimmune tendencies are often made worse by wheat or gluten. Gluten can disrupt the gut lining and cause inflammation in many parts of the body. By balancing her gut microbiome, she could resolve her sugar cravings, skin issues, and headaches.

Her nervous system is off balance because of her neck injury, and stress is causing additional head and neck tension. This affects the function of her vagus nerve, a major factor in the function of the organs of digestion. The vagus nerve is a key nerve that transports information to and from the gut and brain. If the vagus nerve is out of balance, then digestion can easily be affected.

After reading this book and working through the gut reset protocol, Jamie feels like herself again. She feels empowered that she was able to effect change through diet and lifestyle choices. Since the gut reset, she has only one cold, and it was short and mild.

She loves the emotional regulation skills she has learned. She and the children practice them together before bed. She saw her daughter, Sarah, practicing one before an exam one morning to calm the butterflies in her stomach.

Jamie's increase in energy motivates her to do some deep cleaning. She decides to clean out her closet. She is pleasantly surprised when she fits into some favourite clothes she'd shoved to the back of the closet—two sizes smaller than the ones she wore six months ago. She's dropped 15 pounds and feels great in these outfits. When she looks in the mirror, she notices her skin glows. She took a course of supplements and is now on a maintenance routine to keep her microbiome happy. She has energy to be active through the week and no longer has to scout out where all the bathrooms are when she goes out. Weekends at the cottage with her family are rejuvenating, and she is more aware of clean water consumption.

She is more receptive to Rob's advances, which seem to be more frequent lately. Jamie feels like her younger self, and Rob feels like his.

MEET ROB

Rob is a 40-year-old married male with two children—one from his wife, Jamie's, first marriage, and one of their own. He figures he has adult attention deficit disorder (ADD) and has read on the internet that regular physical activity might help him manage his condition. So he took up baseball. At first, he really looked forward to games. But lately, he's noticed that when he runs the bases, he feels like he is tripping over himself. He attributes this to maybe a little arthritis, stress, and lack of physical activity since he's been working more overtime. All this leaves him little time to visit with his parents, and he is concerned about both of them. Dad's memory is slipping, and Mom has to do most of the home care.

Volumes have been down at work, and he is worried about it. They just let another 200 people go, and he's afraid his department will be next on the chopping block. He loves Jamie and tries not to take his stress out on her, but sometimes he just bursts out with anger. He feels guilty for taking things out on her. But that's not all. Lately, his sex drive isn't what it used to be. He's not sure whom to talk to, and he doesn't think Jamie really notices because she's been so consumed with the kids and her work. Rob figures once work settles down, things will get better. But he is scared— what if they don't?

Rob figures he is stressed, but who isn't? He has no idea he has issues related to his gut. He doesn't know the area of his brain that controls coordination reacts to gluten. Other food sensitivities to tomatoes and peppers aggravate his psoriasis and joint pain. The lack of sex drive freaks him out. He doesn't know that inflammation from the gut is affecting his ability to make serotonin and that this contributes to lower testosterone levels and lagging sex drive. To top things off, all the stress has started to interfere with his digestion.

Rob's ADD is a genetic disease, and that means his family, namely his dad and child, are also at risk. In fact, Jamie is run ragged not just from her own problems but also from helping young Johnny deal with his attention-deficit problems in school.

Fast forward, and now after the gut reset and adherence to a gluten-free diet, Rob's knee pain is much better, and his running is back to normal. He even won MVP of his baseball tournament last weekend. He feels coordinated again. His bowels are regular without the use of laxatives for the first time in years. ADD symptoms and blood sugar regulation have improved. His focus and concentration have improved, and he has fewer outbursts of anger. His sex drive isn't what it was at 24, but he is now in the mood much more often than he was before the reset. Now that he understands the genetic component of his gluten intolerance, he is much more patient with his father and realizes how much the two of them are alike. Seeing the lab results in full colour certainly hit him. After a couple of bouts of cross-contamination with gluten, he realizes how much it really bothers his gut and his mood. Outbursts and anger in Rob have reduced but still exist in his dad. It is hard to get Mom to cook gluten-free for his father, but she is more understanding of Rob's preferences and allows him to bring his own pasta for her to cook. And she is careful to let Rob read and coach her on all the ingredients in her homemade sauces so she can cook for her son again.

See how gut health can impact a whole family? With better gut care, new examples are set for generations to come. By peeling back their own personal layers of health, Rob and Jamie make big changes in their lifestyle and diet choices. They learn how to emotionally regulate and better manage their stress.

"Don't judge a man by where he is, because you don't know how far he has come."

—C. S. LEWIS

Whether you have many or just a few issues, this book can help you.

What has brought you to this book?

Here's a snapshot of what's to come:

- Get to the root cause of your health problems
- Identify clues your body gives about your health
- Learn how to create a personalized eating plan
- Become familiar with tests that can evaluate gut health

- Learn tools to support the detoxification process
- Deal with challenges of change
- Support for better sleep (and why it is related to gut health)
- Skills to manage stress (and why it is related to gut health)
- Tune into your inner wisdom—build your core strength
- Maintain your optimum health

What this book is not:

- Professional medical advice
- Meant to diagnose or treat you or any condition you may have
- A cure for anything
- A guarantee for perfect health
- A quick fix

I'm here to help you not just because of my medical training and experience with hundreds of patients, but more so because I have done the hard work to reset my own gut and address health issues that resolved only when my gut senses were fully honoured. After becoming a naturopathic doctor, my journey led me to become a HeartMath® Certified Practitioner so I could learn better skills to regulate my own emotions. I now run programs with patients who come back years later to say how much they still love using the skills! You will learn more about HeartMath® in chapters 8 and 10. I became a level 2 Certified Gluten-Free Practitioner so I could better understand celiac and non-celiac gluten sensitivity; I needed something scientific to explain my many food reactions. This ongoing program is designed and delivered for health professionals by Dr. Tom O'Bryan, www.thedr.com, author of *The Autoimmune Fix* and *You Can Fix Your Brain*. Then I wanted more definitive measures to detect the early signs and development of disease so I wouldn't always be waiting for lab results. I needed something to enrich what I'd learned so I could better apply my knowledge to real, complex cases. That's why I pursued the designation of ADAPT Trained Practitioner from Kresser Institute, the only functional medicine and ancestral health training company. It's a yearlong interactive program with Chris Kresser, www.kresserinstitute.com (author of *The Paleo Cure*, *Your Personal Paleo Diet*, and *Unconventional Medicine*). ADAPT teaches practitioners treatment plans for patients that are highly personalized and based not only on lab results but also on unique genes, lifestyle, health status, and goals.

I am passionate about how we are knit together. And the more patients I deal with, the more research I do, the more I find the root cause of issues is in the gut! It may not be glamourous, but it's worth being aware of.

Are you ready to reset your gut and reset your life? I can't wait to help you! Let's get started.

BACKGROUND: LET'S GET ON THE SAME PAGE

This is the book I needed to write. The first step of my journey was to convince myself with scientific evidence that what I experience is real.

Too often, I sat in doctor's offices, and they looked at me like I had three heads. I don't want that for you.

What I dearly hope this read will give you is increased awareness about the root cause of your health problems. It is designed to empower you to have more productive conversations with your medical support professionals. Although you need answers for the strange sensations you get in your body, they need scientific evidence to represent your case. When you are armed with proper questions, you will get a diagnosis more quickly. A diagnosis isn't the endpoint; it's just a label. But that label can help doctors zero in on the treatment that will help you get better.

Now, before we dive in, you might like to know that GUT is an acronym for gastrointestinal urinary tract. But it also is often referred to simply as the gut (in lowercase), which many people assume to be the contents of their belly. I find that typing GUT in all caps feels like shouting, although you might admit there are plenty of times your GUT shouts at you. Maybe it is doing so right now. Maybe that's why you are reading this book. I'm okay with loud and clear. But I am also here to help you tune into the quieter voice of the gut. To hear what it has to say when it whispers to you. Let's agree to use the lowercase word for ease of reading and learning about the gut.

EMOTIONAL HEALTH AND THE GUT

Early on in humankind's evolution, the gut was our most valued organ. Then, as we became upright citizens, our brains developed more sophisticated processing centres and stole the show.

Your gut is your primary sensing organ. When you sample your environment, you often do so through your digestive tract. I argue that it is not only food we digest. We must also digest the world around us. When this becomes difficult, such as in times of intense or chronic stress, our digestive processes break down.

Anxiety and depression can be symptoms of ill gut health rather than conditions unto themselves. Stay tuned.

What are the common reactions when you experience something beyond your digestive capacity?

Common gastrointestinal symptoms:

- Heartburn
- Indigestion
- Nausea and vomiting
- Diarrhea
- Constipation
- Abdominal pain, bloating, or cramping

Common coexisting mood disorders:

- Anxiety
- Depression
- Attention deficit disorder

Common coexisting conditions related to gut health:

- Cognitive decline
- Eczema
- Rosacea
- Psoriasis
- Rheumatoid arthritis
- SLE/lupus
- Fibromyalgia
- Polymyalgia

- Hypothyroidism
- Autoimmune disease
- Osteoporosis
- Infertility
- Anemia
- Epilepsy and seizures
- Peripheral neuropathy
- Cardiovascular disease
- Diabetes mellitus
- Obesity
- Cancer

Do you experience any of these? You are not alone. Remember Rob and Jamie?

Irritable bowel syndrome can be the result of many factors and can have many symptoms. Typically, it involves frequent changes from loose stools to difficult-to-pass stools. It may also mean going three to five times a day, or not having a bowel movement for days. IBS affects 10–20 percent of the population worldwide. Many don't get the help they need. As you can see, it's not just the bathroom stuff we're talking about. Many people find their health deteriorating and have no idea why.

The microbiome's tasks include detoxification, protection, and regulation of other body systems such as hormone and energy distribution networks, the immune system, and the brain.[3] It also

---

3   Schippa, S., & Conte, M. P. (2014). Dysbiotic events in gut microbiota: Impact on human health. *Nutrients*, 6(12), 5786–5805. https://doi.org/10.3390/nu6125786

provides you nutrients such as folate, vitamin K, biotin, riboflavin (B2), cobalamin (B12), and possibly other B vitamins.[4]

ROLE OF A HEALTHY MICROBIOME

- Fat storage
- Detoxification
- Energy production
- Converts food into available nutrients
- Works with our immune system
- Affects our mood—happy, sad, or depressed
- Produces vitamins
- Reduces inflammation

Microbiome composition varies from person to person. One thousand fifty-seven individual types of microbes have been identified and cultured in the human microbiota. Each of us has our own unique combination of about 160 different micro-organisms.[5,6] They are mostly bacteria but can also include fungi, protozoa, and viruses. Think of the microbiome like your fingerprint: unique.

THIS BOOK MAY SAVE YOU YEARS OF PAIN!

The first part of the book is a straightforward logical exercise

4   LeBlanc, J. G., Milani, C., de Giori, G. S., Sesma, F., van Sinderen, D., & Ventura, M. (2013). Bacteria as vitamin suppliers to their host: A gut microbiota perspective. *Current Opinion in Biotechnology*, 24(2), 160–168. https://doi.org/10.1016/j.copbio.2012.08.005

5   Qin, J., Li, R., Raes, J., Arumugam, M., Burgdorf, K. S., Manichanh, C., Nielsen, T., Pons, N., Levenez, F., Yamada, T., Mende, D. R., Li, J., Xu, J., Li, S., Li, D., Cao, J., Wang, B., Liang, H., Zheng, H., Xie, Y., Wang, J. (2010). A human gut microbial gene catalogue established by metagenomic sequencing. *Nature*, 464(7285), 59–65. https://doi.org/10.1038/nature08821

6   Rajilić-Stojanović, M., & de Vos, W. M. (2014). The first 1000 cultured species of the human gastrointestinal microbiota. *FEMS Microbiology Reviews*, 38(5), 996–1047. https://doi.org/10.1111/1574-6976.12075

supporting my claims with evidence-based medical research. I bring it to life with plenty of patient and personal stories.

In the latter half, we'll use more emotional effort to reach beyond the tangible interface to the glue that binds us—what is not seen but sensed. As I wrote this, I had to trust myself. Trust is a big hurdle for me. Is it for you?

It is up to you what you choose to take or leave. This book is meant to be power under you, to lift you up. Never power over you.

Without help like this book gives you, it may take years of visits to multiple doctors for you to figure out how to feel better. I want more for you. You have a life to live and people around you who need your love!

IT'S NOT YOUR FAULT

Here's what you'll learn in this chapter:

- You didn't know: how food affects the microbiome
- It's not your fault: how North American culture makes gut health difficult
- You didn't know: you have a toxic bucket
- You can't control everything: how you can influence the expression of your genes and how you age
- How to create a timeline to track your health

YOU DIDN'T KNOW

Daphne was on leave from the city for six months. While away, she let her sister use her car. When she came back to reclaim her vehicle, it wasn't in the same shape she left it. Her sister just doesn't care for things the way she does. Upon cleaning it out, she found a sandwich from a nationwide food chain under the driver's seat. Her sister claimed she hadn't been at that food chain in over four months. You'd think it would be stinky and full of mold. It wasn't.

"Disgusting as it may sound," Daphne comments, "it still looked so good you could eat it."

Of course she didn't! But how can this be? The answer is that there are so many preservatives in processed food that it can't even break down after spending four hot months under the seat of a car. That says a lot about whether it can break down in your digestive tract into usable blocks of nutrients. How many meals a day do you eat that are like this sandwich?

Cheese should get moldy. Meat should rot and stink. That's natural. Sometimes bad is good, if you get what I mean.

IT'S NOT YOUR FAULT

It's not your fault. Our culture does not help here. You try to work, raise a family, and look after a home, exercise, and have some time with family and friends. Most people do their best to get to the grocery store to buy some food and maybe cook it. Many just use the drive-through or convenience shopping to pick up a quick snack. You trust that these big chains give you the nourishment you need to get through your day.

These places are businesses, motivated by profit. They make the food as cheap and tasty as they can to keep you coming back for more. What you don't know is that processed and packaged foods (even the packages bought in the grocery store) often contain preservatives to extend shelf life, colouring agents to make it look appealing, and sugar, salt, and bad fats to make you crave it. Trouble is, if a food isn't healthy, fresh, and vibrant, neither are you when you consume it.

I'm guessing you have much more difficult things to digest in your life than a fast food wrap. You are still in the right place. Read on.

FOOD CHANGES THE MICROBIOME

Food affects the gut. Not only does food feed you; it also feeds your microbiome. Food matters: food type, food timing, food quality, food quantity. Foods have enzymes, which are natural body chemicals that take one substance and convert it to another. They help with digestion and nutrient breakdown. Diet is a particular factor in the balance of your gut flora. There are even clear microbiome differences between vegetarians, vegans, and omnivores.[7]

Even food timing makes a difference. Did you know your rhythm and routines can impact your gut health? Hint: it's not just your body that has a biorhythm. Your gut microbes do, too. We will talk about this more in chapter 8.

Food quantity. Did you know that overeating can impact the landscape of the microbiome? It takes most people's guts about six weeks to return to normal after Christmas vacation. Throw in alcohol and too much sugar, and it's a triple whammy.

---

7   David, L. A., Maurice, C. F., Carmody, R. N., et al. (2014). Diet rapidly and reproducibly alters the human gut microbiome. *Nature*, 505(7484), 559–563. https://doi.org/10.1038/nature12820

ORGANIC OR NONORGANIC?

To be or not to be? Organic and non-GMO make a difference. Otherwise, you may ingest glyphosate,[8] herbicides (Roundup®), or pesticides and insecticides that kill the bugs that eat the plants your food grows on. Think of that for a second. If these poisons kill those bugs, will they also kill the bugs in us? Is that a good thing?

Although we are busy trying to feed the masses, we, and our microbes, are dying to eat. Glyphosates alter the microbiome and promote the gram-negative bacteria's release of inflammation-generating toxins. Gram-negative bacteria are disease-generating and can be difficult to control; they have cell walls that are structurally different from gram-positive bacteria, which increase their resistance to the immune system's response, multiple drugs, and antibiotics. This is one reason why the widespread use of pesticides is linked to chronic inflammation, obesity, and disease.[9] The absorption of herbicides like Roundup® is undeniable.[10]

TOXINS AND THE MICROBIOME

Toxic bucket. We all have one. You don't even start with a clean one. At birth, you could have up to 200 environmental chemicals floating around your bloodstream. It's not your fault. It has accumulated over generations before you. Generally, people don't take much notice. They ignore the facts. Toxins are an inevitable

---

8   Rueda-Ruzafa, L., Cruz, F., Roman, P., & Cardona, D. (2019). Gut microbiota and neurological effects of glyphosate. *Neurotoxicology*, 75, 1–8. https://doi.org/10.1016/j.neuro.2019.08.006

9   Liang, Y., Zhan, J., Liu, D., et al. (2019).Organophosphorus pesticide chlorpyrifos intake promotes obesity and insulin resistance through impacting gut and gut microbiota. *Microbiome*, 7(1), 19. https://doi.org/10.1186/s40168-019-0635-4

10   Zocchi, M., & Sommaruga, R. (2019). Microplastics modify the toxicity of glyphosate on Daphnia magna. *The Science of the Total Environment*, 697, 134194. https://doi.org/10.1016/j.scitotenv.2019.134194

part of life. They are a part of your interaction with the world. How do you digest them?

Toxins come from myriad sources:

- Pesticides, herbicides, and insecticides on our food
- Mold and mildew
- Chemicals from manufacturing plants and industrial farms in the air and waterways
- Exhaust from vehicles on the road and boats in the water
- Off-gassing from paints, plastics, and other chemicals we might inhale at work or home
- Heavy metals like lead, mercury, and cadmium sneak into our bodies, too. Do you store any food in lead crystal? Do you have mercury tooth fillings?
- Food sensitivities
- Alcohol consumption
- Dust, pollen, animal dander
- Food storage such as plastics, Teflon coating, and lead paint on dishes
- Household cleaners and laundry detergent, dryer sheets
- Personal care products with sodium laureth sulfate, triclosan, fragrance, perfume, BHA, BHT, coal tar dyes, DEA-related ingredients, dibutyl phthalate, formaldehyde- release preservatives, parabens, PEG compounds, petroleum, or siloxanes. Check out https://davidsuzuki.org/queen-of-green/dirty-dozen-cosmetic-chemicals-avoid/ for more information and support.

Emotional stress also builds chemical toxins up in your body. Have you had a major stressor such as abuse, trauma, job change, moving, death, divorce, or a natural disaster hit you in the last six months? Day to day, how do you digest the world around you? Do you find it "tough to swallow"? Do you have trouble finding the "gall" to make decisions? If we are not emotionally digesting our life, our digestive tract takes a direct hit.

I'll bet you didn't know there was plastic in your diet. One study examined the levels of plastic in human feces (poop) from people all over the world. What did they find? Higher levels of microplastics than found in the contaminated oceans. Do you store food in plastic? Use plastic wrap? Heat in the microwave in plastic? Leave a plastic water bottle in the hot car or freezer? Drink out of plastic cups? Styrofoam cups? Put a plastic lid on your to-go coffee or tea? Use those cute triangle teabags? Do you have a plastic dental retainer in your mouth? Yep. It's all plastic. As it turns out, paper, glass, and stainless steel are safer bets for food storage.

Ingestion of plastics can not only come from food storage but also food itself. Discarded plastic waste enters waterways to the tune of eight million metric tons per year.[11] Sad for our oceans. Sad for us, too: it comes back to haunt us through consumption of fish, mussels, and even through contamination of watersheds servicing local livestock farms. Regardless of the origin of your plastic exposure, it disrupts your microbiome.[12]

Plastics are known endocrine disrupters, meaning they mess with your hormones. They also contribute to nerve damage. There is a

---

11 Rhodes, C. J. (2018). Plastic pollution and potential solutions. *Science Progress, 101*(3), 207–260. https://doi.org/10.3184/003685018X15294876706211

12 Wright, S. L., & Kelly, F. J. (2017). Plastic and human health: A micro issue? *Environmental Science & Technology, 51*(12), 6634–6647. https://doi.org/10.1021/acs.est.7b00423

significant link observed between urine BPA (plastic) levels and both cardiovascular disease and type 2 diabetes.[13]

Plastic can contribute to gastrointestinal inflammation, changes in fat and energy metabolism, higher levels of oxidative stress, and less variety of healthy bacteria in the gut, which has been linked to inflammatory bowel disease.

Inflammation has a complex interrelated relationship with hormonal imbalance. A healthy diversity of the gut microbiota is required for the normal development of the hypothalamic-pituitary-adrenal (HPA) stress axis. When the microbiome is out of order, it contributes to irritability, anxiety, and stress.

What can you do to lessen the impact of toxins on your life?

There is no question we are swimming in a sea of toxins. The bigger questions are: (1) How can you reduce your toxic burden? and (2) How enabled is your body to detoxify? There is a handout at the end of the book to help you with daily detox. It's not something you do once in a while. Your body does it all the time. Your gut is a big part of the process, since you meet a large percentage of your environment through your gut.

ALCOHOL

Alcohol in high doses is a toxin to all cells. If your body is always

---

13   Melzer, D., Rice, N. E., Lewis, C., Henley, W. E., & Galloway, T. S. (2010). Association of urinary bisphenol a concentration with heart disease: Evidence from NHANES 2003/06. *PloS One*, 5(1), e8673. https://doi.org/10.1371/journal.pone.0008673

trying to detox from alcohol, it has little chance to detox from anything else.

Alcohol induces changes to the gut microbiome composition and may be associated with inflammation in the gut, disruption to the gastrointestinal lining, and if persistently consumed to excess, liver disease.

Did you know your body can brew its own alcohol? There is something called autobrewery syndrome (ABS), whereby an imbalanced gut microbiome can ferment its own alcohols after consumption of a carbohydrate-rich meal. ABS is linked to yeast infections (overgrowth of yeast). Just like yeast ferments wine or beer, it can ferment things in your gut, too. Imagine getting a buzz off a bagel. With ABS, that's entirely possible.

Do you experience gas, pain, bloat, headache, joint pain, or feeling hungover without the party? These are all symptoms of ABS. But fungus and yeast are not always to blame. There are alcohol-producing bacteria such as *Klebsiella pneumonia*. Interestingly enough, it is found in higher amounts in those with nonalcoholic fatty liver disease.[14]

Alcohol is not all bad in healthy people. Drinking red wine once every two weeks is enough to achieve a more diverse and healthier gut microbiome.[15] Not so with white wine, beer, or spirits

---

14   Yuan, J., Chen, C., Cui, J., Lu, J., Yan, C., Wei, X., Zhao, X., Li, N., Li, S., Xue, G., Cheng, W., Li, B., Li, H., Lin, W., Tian, C., Zhao, J., Han, J., An, D., Zhang, Q., Wei, H.,...Liu, D. (2019). Fatty liver disease caused by high-alcohol-producing *Klebsiella pneumoniae*. *Cell Metabolism, 30*(4), 675–688.e7. https://doi.org/10.1016/j.cmet.2019.08.018

15   Le Roy, C. I., Wells, P. M., Si, J., Raes, J., Bell, J. T., & Spector, T. D. (2020). Red wine consumption associated with increased gut microbiota α-diversity in 3 independent cohorts. *Gastroenterology, 158*(1), 270–272.e2. https://doi.org/10.1053/j.gastro.2019.08.024

consumption. This may be the link red wine has to lower levels of obesity and "bad" (LDL) cholesterol: it contains polyphenols, which are high in antioxidants and contribute to better health.

If you do drink, be wise. Drink no more than one glass per day for women or two for men and not every day. Also, give your body extended vacations from it now and then. If you always fill yourself with alcoholic spirits, you leave little room for the Holy and Divine Spirit to fill your soul.

INFECTION AND THE MICROBIOME

Over half of the people with IBS have small intestinal bacterial overgrowth (SIBO[16] and about 20 percent of the time, gastrointestinal infection of any sort will result in long-term IBS.[17]

There's a reason over 70 percent of your immune system is in your gastrointestinal tract. It's where you meet a lot of intruders. This is where your frontline forces are doing their best to ward off entry from our environment, while at the same time working to allow nutrients to flow into your body. It makes sense that this process is very selective, much like crossing the border between countries. Passport, please.

Toxins include bacteria, yeast, fungus, protozoa, parasites, spirochetes, worms, and prions. Have you ever had an infection?

---

16 Ford, A. C., Spiegel, B. M., Talley, N. J., & Moayyedi, P. (2009). Small intestinal bacterial overgrowth in irritable bowel syndrome: Systematic review and meta-analysis. *Clinical Gastroenterology and Hepatology*, 7(12), 1279-1286. https://doi.org/10.1016/j.cgh.2009.06.031

17 Spiller, R., & Garsed, K. (2009). Infection, inflammation, and the irritable bowel syndrome. *Digestive and Liver Disease*, 41(12), 844-849. https://doi.org/10.1016/j.dld.2009.07.007

Food poisoning? Then you may harbour one or more of these unwelcome guests.

Mold and mildew can get into the body and complicate things. Check at home, cottage, work, or where you spend most of your day. Windowsills, basements, and bathrooms are the worst offenders. Look for white or black mold, rotten drywall, and water-damaged floors, walls, or woodwork. All are telltale signs of water damage. Where there is water damage, there is susceptibility to mold. Mold is a fungus, and these guys like to hang out in dark, moist places. That includes your gut!

Yeast can convert into fungi. *Candida spp.* is a common yeast that naturally occurs in your gut. For many reasons, it can overgrow, and plenty of health concerns, including other fungal infections, are related to *Candida* overgrowth.

What gets onto our food from dirty hands or dirty water can also make us sick. How many people don't wash their hands after going to the bathroom? My husband once told me a story of a morning at the gym. Guys are in the sauna; one exits to go to the bathroom. A close-the-door, #2 bathroom visit. Through the sauna window, it was obvious this grown man went to the bathroom, had a poo, and returned to the sauna without even washing his hands. No soap, no water. Nada. Eew.

E. coli is one of the top pathogens transmitted by dirty bathroom hands and is related to food poisoning. Now everything Mr. Dirty Hands touches will potentially get poop on it. Imagine this guy in the restaurant where he works. He goes to the bathroom there. He still doesn't wash or doesn't wash properly. Guess what ends up in the food you eat? Not only does *E. coli* make you sick for a number of days, but it can permanently alter your microbiome.

Foodborne pathogens like salmonella can be in undercooked food or be spread through cross-contamination of raw meat juices onto utensils or uncooked food. These are just two examples. Food poisoning can be from bacteria, virus, parasite, molds, toxins, or allergens. Symptoms include a sore tummy, diarrhea, nausea, vomiting, fever, and dehydration.

The key to avoid food poisoning is to properly store, cook, clean, and handle foods.[18]

LYME DISEASE

Did you grow up in, or have you visited, a tick-infested area? Do you know if you have ever had a tick bite? Camping, hiking, cross-country running, outdoor parks, and recreation all increase your exposure. Lyme disease from a tick bite could be the cause of your nausea, diarrhea, or constipation.

Intestinal pseudo-obstruction (stool blockage/constipation) can be a part of the Lyme disease experience. The bowel acts as if it is blocked, but the real culprit is the inflammation and shock to the immune system in response to the spirochete. Care for the gut, and ultimately the immune system, is critical to recovery from a Lyme infection. If you have chronic constipation unexplained by any other factors and live in or have visited an area where ticks are prevalent, it is best to include this in your list of potential root causes of gut problems.

---

18 https://www.niddk.nih.gov/health-information/digestive-diseases/food-poisoning/treatment, accessed March 10, 2020.

INFLUENZA AND OTHER VIRUS INVASIONS

Influenza, Norwalk virus, or any other viral load you ingest will first be met by the mucosal immune system in the gut. Needless to say, when you send your troops to war, there will be casualty. It will take time to rebuild the forces and may need some reinforcement (probiotics, prebiotics) to do so.

PARASITES

Parasites live off their host (you) and have the potential to cause damage such as inflammation and leaky gut. Parasites are passed around through contaminated food and water, day care centres, foreign travel, mosquitoes, pests, pets, and sexual interactions. If there are symptoms, they are usually diarrhea, mucus, blood in the stool, fever, irregular bowel movement, and stomach pain. Parasites can also cause joint pain, skin rashes, allergic reactions, a weakened immune system, and fatigue.

Samantha and Paul

Samantha is a regular patient of mine. She is very proactive in her and her family's health and well-being. Because she's had chronic sinus congestion and an irritated eye, Samantha completed a stool analysis a couple of months ago and found she has an overgrowth of *Candida* and some organisms in her microbiome that are out of balance. We did the gut reset protocol and expect to test again in a few months. With the treatment, her eyes and sinuses are healthy again.

Then Paul, her husband, comes to see me. If the healthiest person he knows (his wife) has a gut imbalance, what's going on in *his* gut?

He doesn't admit to any symptoms. Maybe his experience is his normal. This is often the case. Patients don't necessarily lie about their health; they just aren't sure what's normal and what's not.

The report tells me his samples are loose and watery. That means diarrhea. There are no inflammatory factors and nothing indicating a leaky gut. Good, we may have caught it in time. The test results find he has a parasite, *Dientamoeba fragilis*. This parasite may or may not cause symptoms in adults, whereas in 90 percent of affected children, it does. Usually, it causes noninvasive diarrhea. It can be found in people worldwide. Paul travels for business and has young children at home. He could have picked up the parasite from travel or a pinworm infestation the children brought home from the day care. The children were treated last November, but he thought he was fine.

Our battles are truly in the realm of what we cannot see.

Paul is now on a parasite cleanse, a professional formula I use that includes wormwood, black walnut, aloe, garlic, goldenseal root, quassia, grapefruit seed extract, clove, oregano oil, and sage leaf. Plus, he will take a probiotic suited for IBS. We'll retest within six months to ensure the parasite is gone. Note that what is right for Paul may not be right for you. Please consult your medical provider before starting a course of treatment.

MEDICATION AFFECTS THE MICROBIOME

Medications are supposed improve our health. Sometimes they can be obstacles. There are numerous medications that affect the microbiome. I bet you didn't know that. It's not your fault.

There's more. It's not just individual drugs that alter the microbiome; there is a compound effect. When someone takes more than five drugs, there is a reduction in the overall healthy types of flora and an increase in troublesome bacteria such as *H. pylori*. or *C. difficile*. Additionally, when someone is on any particular drug(s), their gut favours those microbes that are required to metabolize (break down) the drugs.[19]

Drugs can also contain allergens, such as gluten. For those who are really sensitive, a good website is www.glutenfreedrugs.com, or check with your pharmacist. Nonmedicinal components of the drugs are linked to changes in the microbiome—namely, polyethylene glycol (PEG), which is used in solubilizing agents, tablet binders, plasticizers in film coating, and tablet lubricants.[20]

I understand that sometimes drugs can be very helpful. But be aware. If you aren't on any meds, chances are, someone you love is.

DRUGS THAT AFFECT THE MICROBIOME

Many medications disrupt the natural flora and damage the gut lining. Those with antibacterial actions, such as antibiotics, certain cancer therapies, antihistamines, antipsychotics, antihy-

---

19 Ticinesi, A., Milani, C., Lauretani, F., Nouvenne, A., Mancabelli, L., Lugli, G. A., Turroni, F., Duranti, S., Mangifesta, M., Viappiani, A., Ferrario, C., Maggio, M., Ventura, M., & Meschi, T. (2017). Gut microbiota composition is associated with polypharmacy in elderly hospitalized patients. *Scientific Reports, 7*(1), 11102. https://doi.org/10.1038/s41598-017-10734-y

20 D'Souza, A. A., & Shegokar, R. (2016). Polyethylene glycol (PEG): A versatile polymer for pharmaceutical applications. *Expert Opinion on Drug Delivery, 13*, 1257–1275.

pertensives, and SSRIs,[21] are particularly damaging. Sometimes changes are reversed after the patient stops taking the drug, but damage can persist for up to four years.[22] Meanwhile, other medications not only affect the microbiome; they can cause other complications as well.

MEDICATION	POTENTIAL EFFECTS
Antidiabetic drugs (Metformin)	Gut disruption could contribute to risk of additional autoimmune disease.
Proton pump inhibitors (PPIs) Drugs ending in "-azole": Prevacid, Nexium, Dexilant, Prilosec	Contributes to lowered stomach acid, decreased enzyme release, B12 deficiency, and poor digestion. Causes polymicrobial small bowel bacterial overgrowth (SIBO). Linked with celiac disease and *C. difficile* diarrheal infection.[23] Contributes to bacterial resistance to antibiotics, including vancomycin (often used in antibiotic-resistant infections).[24]
NSAIDs (nonsteroidal anti-inflammatory drugs) Advil, Motrin (ibuprofen), Aspirin, Celebrax (celecoxib), Cambia, Voltaren-XR, Zipsor, Zorvolex (dicolofenac), or Idocin (indomethacin)	Ongoing use and administration without food causes bleeding, inflammation, and ulceration in the stomach and small intestine.

21 Munoz-Bellido, J. L., Munoz-Criado, S., & Garcia-Rodriguez, J. A. (2000). Antimicrobial activity of psychotropic drugs: Selective serotonin reuptake inhibitors. *International Journal of Antimicrobial Agents, 14*, 177–180.

22 Walsh, J., Griffin, B. T., Clarke, G., & Hyland, N. P. (2018). Drug-gut microbiota interactions: Implications for neuropharmacology. *British Journal of Pharmacology, 175*(24), 4415–4429. https://doi.org/10.1111/bph.14366

23 Freedberg, D. E., Lebwohl, B., & Abrams, J. A. (2014). The impact of proton pump inhibitors on the human gastrointestinal microbiome. *Clinics in Laboratory Medicine, 34*(4), 771–785. https://doi.org/10.1016/j.cll.2014.08.008

24 Willems, R. P. J., van Dijk, K., Ket, J. C. F., & Vandenbroucke-Grauls, C. M. J. E. (2020). Evaluation of the association between gastric acid suppression and risk of intestinal colonization with multidrug-resistant microorganisms: A systematic review and meta-analysis. *JAMA Internal Medicine, 180*(4), 561–571. https://doi.org/10.1001/jamainternmed.2020.0009

MEDICATION	POTENTIAL EFFECTS
Antidepressants	Causes subsequent weight gain. SSRIs increase the small intestine motility rate (more bathroom visits). Tricyclic antidepressants (TCAs) delay gastric emptying (feeling of fullness, perhaps reduced bathroom visits).
Opioids Tylenol #3 with codeine, meperidine (Demerol) morphine, oxycodone (OxyContin), hydrocodone (Vicodin) cocaine, methadone, heroin, and synthetic opioids such as fentanyl	Constipation, nausea, vomiting, bloating In the long term, can actually *cause* pain. Gut barrier dysfunction can lead to multiple food sensitivities and chronic inflammatory patterns such as headaches, joint pain, brain fog, and increased risk of infectious disease.
Birth control pill, hormone replacement therapy	Depletes folic acid, vitamins B2, B6, B12, C, and E, and the minerals magnesium, selenium, and zinc. Gastrointestinal inflammation.[25] Increases the risk of developing Crohn's disease by 50 percent.[26] Increases risk of vaginal infection such as bacterial vaginosis, *Trichonomiasis vaginalis*, and *Candida albicans* (yeast) infections. These infections happen most during initial use of the contraceptive pill. It is believed the occurrence goes down over time.[27]
Levothyroxine	Increases risk of small intestinal bacteria overgrowth (SIBO).[28]

25   Khalili, H. (2016). Risk of inflammatory bowel disease with oral contraceptives and menopausal hormone therapy: Current evidence and future directions. *Drug Safety*, *39*(3), 193-197. https://doi.org/10.1007/s40264-015-0372-y

26   Cornish, J. A., Tan, E., Simillis, C., Clark, S. K., Teare, J., & Tekkis, P. P. (2008). The risk of oral contraceptives in the etiology of inflammatory bowel disease: A meta-analysis. *The American Journal of Gastroenterology*, *103*(9), 2394-2400. https://doi.org/10.1111/j.1572-0241.2008.02064.x

27   Rezk, M., Sayyed, T., Masood, A., & Dawood, R. (2017). Risk of bacterial vaginosis, *Trichomonas vaginalis* and *Candida albicans* infection among new users of combined hormonal contraception vs LNG-IUS. *The European Journal of Contraception & Reproductive Health Care*, *22*(5), 344-348. https://doi.org/10.1080/13625187.2017.1365835

28   Brechmann, T., Sperlbaum, A., & Schmiegel, W. (2017). Levothyroxine therapy and impaired clearance are the strongest contributors to small intestinal bacterial overgrowth: Results of a retrospective cohort study. *World Journal of Gastroenterology*, *23*(5), 842-852. https://doi.org/10.3748/wjg.v23.i5.842

On a positive note, the antidepressant Sertraline reduces the impact and growth of Candida species of fungus[29] (that's a good thing).

So many things are not your fault—until you know better. You can't control everything. Let's talk about that now.

YOU CAN'T CONTROL EVERYTHING
GENES

You can't pick your genes. Half from your mom. Half from your dad. The combination of what you get is a lottery. When the big human genome project began, scientists hoped to solve all human health problems. Although helpful to know, our genetic code is not our destiny. True, you can't control which genes you get, but their expression can be impacted by things you have some control over, such as your environment, where you live, what you eat, and how you sleep.

Genetics can play a role in how well a person maintains their microbiome levels. The FUT2 gene is one example. People with alterations to this gene have difficulty holding a steady population of microbes in their gut. You can find out your FUT2 status if you run your 23andme results through Sterling's app on MTH-FRsupport.com or most nutrigenomics engines. I did, and I have found issues with the gene. Even though I know this is not a great hand to be dealt, now I can take extra precaution to support my gut with probiotics in my food and supplement and also do my

---

29   Lass-Florl, C., Ledochowski, M., Fuchs, D., Speth, C., Kacani, L., Dierich, M. P., et al. (2003). Interaction of sertraline with *Candida* species selectively attenuates fungal virulence in vitro. *FEMS Immunology and Medical Microbiology*, 35, 11–15.

best to feed my microbes. My belly is like a bowl with lots of pet goldfish that need to be fed every day.

AGING AND THE MICROBIOME

The composition of your microbiome drastically changes as you grow older. You cannot control your age. But you do have some control over *how* you age.

NEWBORN

It wasn't up to you (and maybe not even up to your mother) if you were born vaginally or by cesarean (C-section). However, far too many mothers are opting for unnecessary C-sections, and that is not so good. Why? An expectant mother's vagina becomes rich with *Lactobacillus* in preparation for the fetus. Its purpose is to inoculate the baby's microbiome during the birth process.

There are studies exploring whether we are born with a clean slate or have a microbiome in utero. Many microbiome species have been detected in the umbilical cord, fetal membrane, and amniotic fluid suggest that a baby in utero may not be totally sterile.[30] If a newborn is delivered by C-section, then the majority of microbes inoculating the baby are those of the delivery room. Talk about scary. These places are not totally sterile and harbour many species that are disadvantageous to ingest. In some hospitals, they will swab the baby with cultures from the mother, but there is nothing like the real deal.

---

30 Jiménez, E., Marín, M. L., Martín, R., Odriozola, J. M., Olivares, M., Xaus, J., Fernández, L., & Rodríguez, J. M. (2008). Is meconium from healthy newborns actually sterile? *Research in Microbiology*, 159(3), 187–193. https://doi.org/10.1016/j.resmic.2007.12.007

The newborn gastrointestinal lining is highly permeable. That means it is fragile and allows most nutrients through without question. That's because the immune system of a newborn needs time to develop. Colostrum, the first product of breast milk, reduces inflammation, protects against irritation and infection, and promotes the repair of the lining. Colostrum is not yet available in formulas, although they are working on it. Still, bottle-fed babies are at a disadvantage.

Another way we gain early access to our microbes is by the touch of skin—there is a microbiome there, too. A baby lying on the mother's skin will incorporate some of her microbiome. Breastmilk also helps build the immune system and the microbiome. Its composition changes as a baby's needs change. It changes with the time of day (more fat content early in the morning) and even day to day and month to month. IgA, part of the immune system, is provided through breastmilk. IgA coats the intestinal lining and protects the mucosal surfaces against infection. This can't happen with formula.

TODDLER

Your microbiome continues to shape and develop itself until you reach the age of 3.[31] Then it appears to level off.[32] Where you live makes a difference. Children raised in the country versus the city, farm or no farm, pets or no pets—factors like these make

---

31 Nuriel-Ohayon, M., Neuman, H., & Koren, O. (2016). Microbial changes during pregnancy, birth, and infancy. *Frontiers in Microbiology, 7,* 1031.https://doi.org/10.3389/fmicb.2016.01031

32 Stark, P. L., & Lee, A. (1982). The microbial ecology of the large bowel of breast-fed and formula-fed infants during the first year of life. *Journal of Medical Microbiology, 15*(2), 189–203. https://doi.org/10.1099/00222615-15-2-189

your microbiome unique.[33] If you move, your microbiome can shift, too. One study found people who emigrated to the United States experienced immediate loss of native strains, which were replaced with US-associated microbiome strains and functions.[34]

ELDERLY

Aging for most means progression to inflammation and reduced immune capacity. Did you know that adverse changes in the microbiome contribute to 16–18 percent of worldwide cancer?

However, a study showed that those who live more than a hundred years have microbiomes that reflect the body's capacity to digest proteins and respond well to inflammation.[35] Watch for news on probiotics that fight aging! Early studies observe how certain microbiome species can take polyphenols from our diet and use them to interfere with the misfolding of proteins. Misfolded protein is one of the key markers of Alzheimer's disease.[36] Want to get a head start? Polyphenols are found in plant-based

33   Yatsunenko, T., Rey, F. E., Manary, M. J., Trehan, I., Dominguez-Bello, M. G., Contreras, M., Magris, M., Hidalgo, G., Baldassano, R. N., Anokhin, A. P., Heath, A. C., Warner, B., Reeder, J., Kuczynski, J., Caporaso, J. G., Lozupone, C. A., Lauber, C., Clemente, J. C., Knights, D., Knight, R., Gordon, J. I. (2012). Human gut microbiome viewed across age and geography. *Nature*, *486*(7402), 222-227. https://doi.org/10.1038/nature11053

34   Vangay, P., Johnson, A. J., Ward, T. L., Al-Ghalith, G. A., Shields-Cutler, R. R., Hillmann, B. M., Lucas, S. K., Beura, L. K., Thompson, E. A., Till, L. M., Batres, R., Paw, B., Pergament, S. L., Saenyakul, P., Xiong, M., Kim, A. D., Kim, G., Masopust, D., Martens, E. C., Angkurawaranon, C.,…Knights, D. (2018). US immigration westernizes the human gut microbiome. *Cell*, *175*(4), 962-972.e10. https://doi.org/10.1016/j.cell.2018.10.029

35   Biagi, E., Candela, M., Fairweather-Tait, S., Franceschi, C., & Brigidi, P. (2012). Aging of the human metaorganism: The microbial counterpart. *Age*, *34*(1), 247-267. https://doi.org/10.1007/s11357-011-9217-5

36   Wang, D., Ho, L., Faith, J., Ono, K., Janle, E. M., Lachcik, P. J., Cooper, B. R., Jannasch, A. H., D'Arcy, B. R., Williams, B. A., Ferruzzi, M. G., Levine, S., Zhao, W., Dubner, L., & Pasinetti, G. M. (2015). Role of intestinal microbiota in the generation of polyphenol-derived phenolic acid mediated attenuation of Alzheimer's disease β-amyloid oligomerization. *Molecular Nutrition & Food Research*, *59*(6), 1025-1040. https://doi.org/10.1002/mnfr.201400544

foods and beverages—notably, apples, berries, citrus fruit, plums, broccoli, cocoa, tea, and coffee.[37] Yum!

SUMMARY OF THINGS THAT AFFECT YOUR MICROBIOME

- Birth process
- Breast or bottle
- Where you grow up
- Infections
- Alcohol
- Drugs
- Plastics
- Chemicals
- Food—timing, quantity, quality, organic, GMO
- Genes
- Aging
- Sleep

It is not your fault if you didn't know these things. Now you do.

"Oh, what a tangled web we weave when at first we practice to deceive."

—SIR WALTER SCOTT, 1808

TIMELINE

What are the main problems you are trying to fix? When did these problems begin? Often, it helps to create a timeline of your life. You can find a timeline template in the appendix. How was your

---

37 Williamson, G. (2017). The role of polyphenols in modern nutrition. *Nutrition Bulletin*, 42(3), 226–235. https://doi.org/10.1111/nbu.12278

mother's health when she was pregnant with you? Her labour? Were there antibiotics or other drugs given? Were you born vaginally or by C-section? Put these details down and then add the date. Where did you live in the first few years of life? On a farm? In the city? What country? Do you know much of your ancestors' or genetic background? Surgeries or trauma? Family medical history? All these things can contribute to the early development of the microbiome.

What's your next milestone?

Did you receive multiple courses of antibiotics as a child? Did you get sick frequently? Any diagnoses such as celiac, constipation, or diarrhea? What about experiences at school? Did you enjoy it? Did you get good grades easily, or did you work hard or hardly work? Why? Put these along the line and write the date.

Add in a section for your teen years. Any illness or major impacts of stress on your life? Write these in.

Continue this decade by decade until you come to your current age. Hold on to this timeline. If you are like me, after a bad health experience, you want to forget all about it. But making a timeline helps put things into perspective.

You might feel a little overwhelmed right now. Even a little defeated. Allow it. Accept it. Sit with it. We aren't meant to live in a bubble where everything is perfect. We all have a toxic bucket. Look at ways you can reduce what you put into it and find ways to drain some out. It might take a while to find a level that is more manageable.

Go slow. Give yourself time to recognize where you have room for improvement. You are peeling back the layers. We need to do this in stages. While you make efforts to implement new habits, also be sure to engage in some creative task: garden, listen to some music, walk in nature, colour, or breathe and meditate.

When you are ready, come on back, and we will listen to what the body has to say. Your body truly speaks for itself.

2

THE BODY SPEAKS FOR ITSELF

Here's what you'll learn in this chapter:

- Peel into the physical layer, the outer layer of the onion
- How to listen to your gut
- The importance of letting go
- The body scan: clues and cues your body gives about gut health

LISTEN TO YOUR GUT

Recently, I attended a professional development course. It was held over two different days six months apart. This course teaches how to listen with fingers. Literally, we place our hands on bodies to find out what we feel. There are the obvious things like muscle tension, knots, and some lumps and bumps. Stay a little longer, and we find organs in the belly twisted and turned. Sometimes valves are stuck open or perhaps the stomach has some fibrous tissue nestling its neck up to the rib cage. We learn to feel for this and release it. The instructor says to me, "*How are you digesting life?*" I think, "Funny, I'd told the group I essentially help people digest their food and the world around them, and here she is asking *me* how I digest life." It makes me wonder. How *do* I digest life? What does she mean by this? I don't ask, but the question sticks with me.

I return six months later for another module of the course. As an eager volunteer, I lay belly up on the table. The instructor zeros in on the top of my stomach again. She asks again, "*How are you digesting life?*" This time, I ask her what she means by that. "*You know,*" she says, "*are you taking things in, using what you need and letting what you don't go?*" Hmm. I am probably missing something here because I still have food sensitivities and am on a bit of a mission to see if I can change that with a microbiome or lifestyle cleanup. Change it at an emotional level and keep the brain sharp. Include the spiritual level. I have been at this for years. Just when I think, "That's it, I've got it—everything will get better now," I am wrong. Well, not all wrong, but not all right yet either. What am I not letting go? Is this part of it?

When there are issues like constipation, I always ask, "What in life are we not letting go?" I am perfectly human, meaning what I do is not perfect, so it's likely there is something of which I am not letting go. But I have no clue what that is. I can be blind to my shadows. You can, too.

Skip forward to a networking event the following week. It is a room full of people in the caring-for-others industry. Caring for aging parents, caring for the caregivers—that kind of business. Not one but three companies are there to represent personal organizing. These companies help people go through their STUFF and figure out what is useful or meaningful and what has got to go. This is a real-deal business. Thank God, because I need them. We have issues with STUFF in our house, as do many in our society. There are local hoarding support groups for people with issues giving up their stuff.

I buy a book called *Buried in Treasures*. (I know, buying more stuff!) I learn how to speak and coach my family members around managing their stuff. Then at home, I clean out my bookshelves and storage. I take some time to unload some of my STUFF, much of which is cookbooks I can't use anymore because they are full of recipes with gluten, dairy, and sugar. Ugh, how symbolic this is! We all hold on to stuff for emotional reasons, and not all of it is in a box or on a bookshelf. Some of it is in our body, like the instructor sensed when she worked with me. Later in the book, we will talk more about this, how it affects your gut, and what you can do about it.

I have spent years working on this personally before I began doing so professionally. I have a sense of what it is like to be in your shoes—to some extent anyway. I am not you. You are not me. We both have a body and a mind and a soul. And a digestive problem (or two) and some anxiety with low mood at times.

Let's see what we can tease apart so we can figure out what's going on and learn the steps to take better care of ourselves. I assure you, as you do this, the rest of your world will become easier to digest. What you'll find in this book is by no means the perfect solution for everyone, but it is a helpful start for many.

Sometimes your body whispers at you.

Other times it screams.

If you aren't digesting your food properly, it can cause all sorts of deficiencies and inflammatory damage to the rest of your body.

"Illnesses do not come upon us out of the blue. They are developed from small daily sins against Nature. When enough sins have accumulated, illnesses will suddenly appear."

—HIPPOCRATES

A big part of what I do is help people understand their bodies. For goodness sake, we have one in a lifetime, and quite frankly, I don't think we take much notice on how to care for it. People spend more time and money on their cars and pets than on the bodies they live in. Most of us walk around like a bunch of talking heads with no connection to the body whatsoever.

You live in your body day in and day out. Twenty-four hours a day, seven days a week. For what? Thirty, forty, fifty, or (hopefully) many more years? I will see you for an hour up front, and then maybe half an hour a week for a few weeks, and the appointments will spread out. You are responsible for you. I am here to teach you more about you.

You may want to grab a notepad to jot down your findings.

"The greatest medicine of all is teaching people how not to need it."

—HIPPOCRATES

Health is a process of evolution, not revolution. Be patient. You didn't end up the way you are overnight. Remember, health is like an onion. It will take time to peel back the layers and rebuild your well-being. We will take it one layer at a time. Begin with the outer layer, the physical. Then emotional, followed by cognitive (clear thinking and good memory), and finally, your spiritual core. Core strength! It means more than abs of steel. Spiritual strength, like our abdominal muscles, is an important stabilizer.

As we go along, observe how you feel, health patterns, past and current environment, exercise routines, sleep habits, diet, and spiritual connection. Continue to build your timeline template as you work through the chapters; it will help give clues to the root cause of what's going on inside of you. What you do today can help you build the stepping stones to tomorrow.

BODY SCAN

It helps to look at yourself. It is amazing how many people don't realize the messages the body will give when you just look at it.

If you do this at home, you can get fully naked to screen yourself. A mirror on the wall and one in your hand will help. You live in your body 24/7, but you won't necessarily understand everything you find. That's normal. Report the details to your doctor at your next visit.

HAIR, SKIN, NAILS

Look at your hair, skin, and nails first. You have to think, why is this important to the health of the gut? Well, hair, skin, and nails are basically protein. If you have low stomach acid and poor nutrient absorption, then you are not breaking down protein as well as you could. This ultimately affects the health of your hair, skin, and nails because they are basically protein. Note the colour and consistency of the hair. Is it thin and limp? Dry? This is a sign of poor nutrient status. If the hair is thick and full of life, then that is a good indication of proper protein and nutrient status. In women, hair growing thick and dark in spots such as the chin, breast, or legs can be a sign of hormonal imbalance. This can have some relation to the gut but indirectly so. Still, note it down.

Look at the scalp—dandruff, flaky, patches of red, scaly? That could be the result of fungal problems, eczema, or psoriasis. These can all start with imbalances in the gut microbiome.

What does the skin tone of your face look like? Can you see changes in areas? Black, grey, blue, or purple is stagnation of energy. Yellow is mild toxicity, and green is strong toxicity. Red is inflammation or trapped anger. White is frozen, lack of energy or blood. You'll see white to clear skin when there is very low iron. Iron is needed to make red blood cells, and good blood circulation is what brings the healthy glow to your cheeks. Black circles under your eyes, even though you've had a decent night's sleep? You could have food sensitivities. If the skin is yellow or the whites of the eyes yellow, we think of jaundice. That means the liver is not detoxifying well or it is overloaded. Yes, the liver is linked to the gut, too. You'll see.

Skin tags can mean insulin dysregulation—that can have a lot to do with your diet and your microbiome. Skin tags are skin-coloured and are like tiny tassels growing off your body. You might find them anywhere, but they often lurk under the arms or chin.

Another breakout? Not only do I hate the terms *zit* and *pimple*, but it's just plain annoying to have a breakout as a grown adult. The most common offenders are dairy and sugar. I got over eating dairy. Okay. But strictly no sugar can, at times, get the best of me. Sometimes I just want to eat some dried apricots or put a little honey in something. Ugh. Busted. Within two days, I'll have bumps on my face. I've even seen gut overgrowth of mold contribute to acne. Treat it, and the acne clears.

Many falsely believe the skin's treatment is only topical. But most of the health comes from the inside out. In fact, great skin is a reflection of a healthy gut. This might make more sense if you understand you are a tube that starts at your mouth and ends at your bum. The skin separates you from the outside world. Even your gastrointestinal tract has a "skin." Its tissue structure is different from the skin on your arm of course, but still, it defines your borders.

Gut skin is very thin—in some places, only one-cell thick. The skin on the soles of your feet is pretty thick, comparatively. Regardless, if you eat something that irritates your skin on the inside, chances are you will see reactions on the skin on the outside.

Rashes. Do you have rashes that come and go? Stick around? What do they look like? Where are they? Conventional medicine labels this "dermatitis" (which just means irritated skin), eczema, psoriasis, or rosacea. These can all start with imbalances in the gut. Also, have you ever gotten clusters of itchy little blisters filled with clear fluid on your arms or legs? These could be viral, could be contact (like from poison oak or ivy), or they just might be from a sensitivity to gluten (dermatitis herpetiformis).

Not everyone with celiac disease gets dermatitis herpetiformis, but if you *do* get it, there's a 99 percent chance you have celiac disease. It can also be a telltale sign if you have been exposed to gluten. I wish my family doctor had followed through on my experience with this. It was early March, so there was no poison ivy or oak around. My shins broke out in tiny little clear fluid-filled blisters. She first thought it was dermatitis herpetiformis, then dismissed it almost immediately. I'm not sure why, but I wish I'd pressed on that. Maybe having a label would help me come to terms with my troubles, although it wouldn't necessarily affect my behavior.

Even "Healthy" Oatmeal Can Be a Pain

"*I challenge you to not eat that oatmeal you brought with you,*" my husband said. We'd just arrived at our tropical vacation spot, and I unpacked a few things in the kitchen. Early in my days of going gluten-free, I was still learning. The oats were steel cut and a good breakfast option. Or so I thought. But it was the last wheat-related grain (a cousin, in fact) still in my diet. And the crusty, red patches behind my right ear and along my chin were not going away. What did I have to lose? I ditched the oats. Damned if my husband, who's no role model when it comes to his diet, was right about mine.

It took three weeks for the rash to subside. That was nothing compared to the three years I'd endured it. Wow. My face was like new again. So was my humility.

Some people have red, beefy rashes in warm moist places like the groin or under the armpits or breasts. *Candida spp.* is a yeast, and when it turns fungal, it can spread body-wide. Since fungi are fun guys, they like to hang out together. Alongside a *Candida* overgrowth, don't be surprised to find tinea. That's athlete's foot, ringworm, and fungal infections of the scalp or beard.

Hydrocortisone cream can help suppress itchy skin, but it does not fix the problem. As soon as you stop applying it, the rash will likely recur. When the gut is inflamed, you are bound to have skin inflammation somewhere. Pay attention. Keep a journal. Get help.

Nancy's Welts

Nancy sure is glad she listened to her body. She is a 24-year-old country-living gal who came in to see me about eighteen months ago. Periodically, for no apparent reason, she would break out in multiple welts that were red, blotchy, and *very itchy*! We identified food sensitivities and reset the gut with botanical antimicrobials, did two rounds of histamine reduction protocol, which included some high doses of B5 and B6, along with six months of high-dose bifido bacteria probiotic. Bifido eats histamine. We now use a curcumin supplement with bromelain and quercetin, a regular probiotic, a 2,000 IU vitamin D3, 1 tablespoon of cod liver oil, B complex vitamin daily, and occasionally Apis 30 C homeopathic, which, taken at early onset can halt the breakout entirely. She is now in maintenance mode—somewhat conscious of what she eats but not always. She has found a protocol she is happy with and feels good living her life. That's what counts.

Unfortunately, six months into maintenance mode, Nancy starts to break out repeatedly, and the symptoms worsen. In addition to all the skin hives, her breathing becomes laboured, and her whole face swells up until she can't even see out of her eyes. I fear an anaphylactic reaction and tell her to get to emergency if this ever happens again. In addition to her protocol, I have her pick up some antihistamine from the pharmacist to take on the way to the hospital in an event. We also make an appointment with her family medical doctor to get a referral to an immunologist. We redo her food sensitivities and eliminate all histamine-based foods from her diet.

A few weeks later, she comes back in looking like a pincushion. The immunologist has tested Nancy for a whole panel of food and environmental items. He hasn't found anything that might have triggered her immune IgE reaction. He's prescribed her some heavy-duty antihistamines, which over the course of three months, Nancy finds helps some but not totally. Eventually, she stops because of the awful abdominal pain that comes as a side effect. We move next to stool analysis. Nancy certainly has *Candida*, but she also has an overgrowth of gram-negative bacteria in her gut, which could be from the farm next door; *Pseudomonas chlororaphis* is often used as a corn crop herbicide. *Blastocystis* parasite and two types of mold are also living in her. The immune IgA lining her gut is low, and her microbiome isn't making enough short-chain fatty acids. This definitely calls for a gut reset. I also check whether she makes immunoglobulins to ensure her immune system is responding. It is! The IgE titers (related to histamine response) are elevated, even while she's taking Blexten, a strong prescriptive antihistamine. After three weeks into parasitic cleanse treatment (described in chapter 5), Nancy feels more energetic and has had zero reactions. We will follow through the gut reset steps to rebalance her microbiome, then work on the repair. Then she can talk to her immunologist about coming off Blexten.

Look Deeply at Any Scars

Other things to look for on the skin are scars. Scars can indicate past trauma, but also scar tissue can make things stick together that were meant to be apart. Scar tissue in the abdominal area may prevent organs of digestion from moving freely. Interestingly enough, sometimes scar tissue in other areas of the body can pull on the areas of the abdomen.

Think of having a T-shirt on and grabbing one of the bottom corners. The whole fabric stretches and tenses up diagonally from the opposite shoulder. The matrix of connective tissue acts in mysterious ways, but if you think of it as fabric you wear, then its behavior is easier to understand. Take note of your visible scar tissue. Think of any operations or other internal scar tissue that might remain. There is an emotional layer to this. Remember the layers? Physical, emotional, cognitive, and spiritual. We are woven together. Knit together. The fabric of your life and your experiences can embed themselves in your flesh and your connective tissue.

Continue with the body scan. After examining your hair and skin, have a look at your nails. The nails tell us quite a bit. Remove your fake nails or nail polish if necessary to get a good look. If you have acrylic nails, then the nails may be damaged by the chemical bonders and removers. Here, we look at natural nails. Thin, brittle, and cracking nails are a sign of poor nutrition or poor absorption. This could mean not enough fats or proteins, or too many simple carbohydrates (sugars) are getting through the gut to your body.

Same goes for vitamin and mineral status. White spotting on the nails, called leukonychia, is a sign of poor calcium, selenium, or zinc status. If only one nail has a spot from something like hitting your nail with the hammer, then that of course is trauma to the nail and not nutritional deficiency. That kind of injury will have to grow out of the nail. These spots tend to go away when the nutrient status in question is restored. Ridges lengthwise or widthwise on the nails can indicate a number of different vitamin or mineral deficiencies. Nails that are curved like a spoon, a condition called koilonychia, could mean deficiency of chromium, iron, selenium, zinc, or vitamins B2, B3, or C.

Fingernails and toenails can also be affected by psoriasis and fungus. Pitting in the nails can mean psoriasis. In this case, your nail looks like a car roof after a hailstorm. The pitting in my nails substantially improved after my gut reset. Autoimmune diseases such as psoriasis can be triggered by poor gut health or leaky gut.

Even the words for toenail fungus sound gross—dermatitis onchymosis or unguium. It is difficult to tell the toenail fungus apart from a bad case of toenail psoriasis. If your toenails are thick, yellow, discoloured, mangy messes, consider asking that a toenail sample be sent to the lab to get a firm diagnosis.

EYES

Pull the lower lids down and see how pink or pale the inside of your eyelids are. This is an area of superfine capillaries and a good place to get an indicator of iron stores. If they are really pink or red, this is a sign of good blood flow and lots of hemoglobin in the blood. A sign of good iron flowing through the bloodstream. If the inner lids are pale, then keep an eye out for other signs of low iron. Is the skin itself pink and rosy? Or is it pale, too? Really pale or translucent skin can be a sign of low iron. If this applies to you, get your iron checked. And ask why your iron might be low. Do you eat red meat? Take a supplement? If you eat red meat or take an iron supplement and you are pale in the skin and conjunctiva (the skin inside the lower eyelids), then what? Well, it means you are not absorbing iron. The reason could be low dietary intake, low stomach acid, poor digestive enzymes from the pancreas to break down the meat fibres, or a disruptive lining of the small intestine that prevents absorption (celiac, Crohn's).

What do the whites of the eyes look like? Are they white? Good. Yellow? Maybe the liver is overburdened. Make notes. Yes, there is a microbiome in the eyes, too.[38] It exists for the purposes of keeping this entry point in the body safe from harmful invaders.

Dry eyes? Even this has links to an inflammatory microbiome.[39]

FACE

Facial markings can provide early warning signs even before blood tests, MRIs, or CT scans detect a problem. A whole record of emotions and experience are held in the lines and contours

38   Lyon, J. (2017). Even the eye has a microbiome. *JAMA, 318*(8), 689. https://doi.org/10.1001/jama.2017.10599

39   Tavakoli, A., & Flanagan, J. L. (2019). The case for a more holistic approach to dry eye disease: Is it time to move beyond antibiotics? *Antibiotics, 8*(3), 88. https://doi.org/10.3390/antibiotics8030088

of the face. Lillian Bridges explains this in her second edition of *Face Reading in Chinese Medicine.* She writes, "I would look at their face and see strength in their colon, but a weakness in their liver." Her client had anger issues, and since their liver was weak, they had to hold the anger somewhere else in their body—that is, their large intestine (colon). The emotion transferred to a stronger organ that could process it. But the large intestine doesn't do so well with anger. Anger needs to be processed and expressed. Instead of sole focus on the colon, some remedies also call for strengthening the liver.

Look at your face. Zero in on the area between the eyes, on the upper bridge of your nose. According to Lillian Bridges, this area on your face represents digestion. Is there a line going from side to side? Not a mark from your glasses, but the place they might fit into. If there is, it means you need to pay attention to your gut and your diet and the enjoyment of your meals in order to make proper energy. Interestingly enough, this line can also mean the ability to digest information in your mind, another piece of evidence that we use similar organs to digest both food and the world around us.

TONGUE

I always get people to stick out their tongue. It's a Chinese medicine thing. It's a conventional medicine thing, too. The tongue body and the tongue coat are both evaluated for health. Organ health is evaluated per the corresponding area on the tongue (see diagram below).

Tongue Body

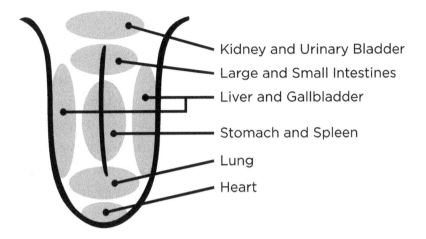

Kidney and Urinary Bladder
Large and Small Intestines
Liver and Gallbladder
Stomach and Spleen
Lung
Heart

The body shape and size of the tongue have meaning. The body gives a sense of what is deep seated, systemic, or chronic. The coat gives clues to more transient, recent imbalances. Thus, the coat will change quickly while the body takes longer to morph.

The general structure of the tongue gives insight into the nutritional status and structural condition of your internal organs. For example, a tongue that is pale is like skin and eye conjunctiva that are pale: it means you should have your iron levels checked.

A tongue should be the right size for the mouth, not too big or too small. Oversized? Perhaps the whole body is in excess. Thin and lacking substance? That likely says weakness in the state of the organs. If the tongue looks like an old country road full of potholes, it's likely because of a lack of digestive enzymes.

Are there cracks going up, down, or sideways? Where? Cracks straight down the centre generally mean stress is affecting digestion. Cracks that go left to right indicate poor organ function. Use the tongue map to see which organ is affected.

What is the colour of the tongue body? A raw, red tongue that looks like a piece of meat is likely telling of deficiency in fluids and general poor nutrition status, especially B vitamin deficiencies. More specifically, a red tip of the tongue can mean B12 deficiency, anxiety, or per Chinese medicine, heat in the heart. People with low B vitamin status are often anxious. You need B vitamins to break down the neurotransmitters of excitement, so if you don't get them, epinephrine and adrenaline hang around too long and you feel anxious.

Tongue Coat

"*My tongue is orange, and I haven't been eating Creamsicles!*" I look at the coat on Sonya's tongue. She says her throat is sore, too. Her trip to Mexico was a disappointment. She had diarrhea, and then when she was back in Canada, the lung issues began with confirmed pneumonia. She was prescribed antibiotics and puffers, which contain cortisone to help the bronchioles open up and to ease laboured breathing.

The downside is that Sonya's system is fragile, and she has a rare long-standing autoimmune disease and history of multiple parasite infestations and food poisoning. I haven't seen her in four months because we had healed her gut to a point that she could enjoy life and manage her health with the routine we'd established. Now, with the courses of antibiotics and puffers, her immune and gut are struggling. What do you think the orange coat means?

After three days of treatment with a botanical antifungal blend, Sonya's tongue coat looks 70 percent better. The plan was to keep on this for a month, but she reacted to the garlic in the formula. We switched to tiny amounts of oil of oregano and cloves, Citracidal®, and a homeopathic *Candida albicans*. Her probiotic is a 500 billion combo of *Lactobacillus* and *Bifidobacterium* intensive-care blend she takes with food at least two hours after the antifungals. She already avoids gluten, sugar, and dairy, so no diet changes are necessary—just rest, lots of steamed green vegetables, and a limit of one fruit per day. She is also on vitamin D3, vitamin C, a B complex, and a calcium-magnesium-potassium tri-salt.

The coat and colour of the body of the tongue give insight into imbalances, especially in the digestive tract. A healthy coat is thin and clear. It glistens a little. What does yours look like? What did you eat recently? Do you smoke? Tobacco can stain the coat on your tongue. So can coffee and red wine. It is best to look first thing in the morning before you brush your teeth or scrape your tongue. Hopefully, you do all that before you do anything else.

If the coat is white, thick, and damp, and it scrapes off easily, then it is likely thrush. Thrush is caused from an overgrowth of *Candida*. Where there is dairy, there is dampness, I always say. *Candida* loves dairy, sugar, and dampness. Most fungi and yeasts like sugary snacks and prefer to live in warm, damp places. If there is a yellow tint to the coat on the tongue, that means heat or inflammation. Orange coat, like Sonja's, can be heat and dampness, too, and still fungal. Damp heat is not so nice. It likely means you'll have diarrhea.

Now you appreciate what the tongue has to say without even

making a peep! The next time someone sticks their tongue out at you, have a good look at it!

While you look in your mouth, check for healthy inner cheeks and gums. Any cankers or sore areas? Jot those down. Remember, the mouth is an area for bacteria to enter. It is also a continuation of the skin and can reflect food sensitivities and imbalances in the gastrointestinal microbiome as well as the local microbiome of the mouth.

Look in your car's rearview mirror (preferably not while driving) and say "Aah." On a bright day, this is a great way to see the uvula (the dangly thing at the back of your mouth). It should hang straight down and go straight up when you say aah. If it goes to the right or left, then there is stress on your vagus nerve. This affects digestion. You will learn how and why in future chapters about how stress and the nervous system relate to the gut.

THE BELLY

What next? Time to listen. What noises does your gut make? Does it rumble a lot? Make gassy fizzles and wind noises? If you put your hands on your tummy, does it feel soft and squishy or tight as a drum? I like to feel around the abdomen and literally listen with my hands and fingers. Both hands and feet can detect vibrations, although I prefer to use my hands (and my patients appreciate that I don't use my feet).

There is a lot going on between the rib cage and the hip bones. Most of your digestive engine is in this area. I feel for consistency of the tissue, placement of organs, lymphatic landscape, connective tissue, scar tissue, valve functioning, stool placement, and consistency. I listen with the stethoscope for gurgling and noises. Sometimes I just hold my fingers or hands over an area and wait for the body to respond. Try it. See for yourself what your belly has to say. Anything? If nothing else, you'll give yourself a real nice tummy massage.

You are well on your way to understanding the physical aspects of gut health and the ways the body tries to tell us what's going on inside. Warning signs, indicators, full-on wagers of war can be seen, heard, and felt. You did a great job observing, recording, looking at, and listening to your body. If you feel a little overwhelmed, that is totally understandable. Not everyone is into discovering how their body is knit together. I just happen to love learning about it. There are so many ways to look at the body, feel it, and observe it.

It's always a good idea to get a medical professional to have a look at you. As we learned here, you can have a grab bag of symptoms with many different causes. Don't discount how and what you feel. It's important. Don't Dr. Google it either. You can educate and empower to ask better questions, but you can't diagnose yourself.

You might feel a little unsure if you find something of concern or even a little frustrated because you want the answers now. After you make notes and book an appointment to see your health professional, take some time to be extremely quiet and deeply attentive. Breathe in and out.

When you are ready, come on back, and we will continue to peel the physical layer of the onion and really appreciate the gut's connection to the rest of your body.

THE GUT CONNECTION

Here's what you'll learn in this chapter:

- How your body works like a team
- Your body is organized in systems, not silos
- Wholistic not hole-istic healthcare
- Dig into digestion
- How the gut connects to the rest of your body

"All disease starts in the gut."

—HIPPOCRATES

I know nothing about hockey. When we go to the local games, I am sure I ask the same questions over and over about what just happened and why the guy is in the penalty box. But I enjoy watching the players chase the puck back and forth on the ice. At times, it allows me to follow thoughts in my mind. Random, ricocheting, persistent thoughts.

I notice differences in how a team plays at the beginning of the season versus the playoffs. Early on, it is quite apparent there are some very good individuals out there on the ice. For the most part, they skate well, shoot well, and defend well. But their timing is off. Emotions get the better of them. When someone passes, he finds his teammate isn't there to take it. Or he misses. They get tripped up by the opposition.

You've seen teams like this. They are good but not great. A great team has synchronicity. After a number of games, they get their groove on. They gel. Instead of a number of individuals skating around on the ice, they are a single cohesive unit acting as one. They flow. Then they score! Maybe even win the game. Occasionally, a player gets hurt. Someone else picks up the position and plays. The team has multiple members who can cover each job, though it is undeniable some individuals are better at specific positions: the guy who plays forward doesn't get put on goal.

Your body is like a hockey team. There are many players working to keep it going. Each plays a designated part. If an organ gets injured, other organs try to take over its duties but may not do such a good job. Get many players injured and the defences are down, and the other team can easily score a goal.

The idea is to see how well your team is playing. Like keeping track of how many assists and goals a player makes in a season. Or how many times they end up in the penalty box.

Your body is constantly on defence. Pathogens such as bacteria, virus, fungi, parasites, spirochetes, and the like greet you through your main contact with the environment, your gastro tract. It starts at the mouth. Your body has defences at other parts, such as your skin barrier, nose, ears, and eyes. As you interact with your environment and go about your day, your body is constantly striving for balance.

Sometimes your body gets overwhelmed. That's when you get symptoms of ill health or disease. If you are quiet enough to listen to your body, you will know what's going on.

"If you are not your own doctor, you are a fool."

—HIPPOCRATES

I like this Hippocrates quote in the sense that we all ought to be responsible for our health. But I also believe you can be a fool if you try to be your own doctor alone.

It takes years to understand the intricate mechanisms of the human body. Scientific research constantly expands and redefines the paradigm of disease and treatments. There is so much to know that no one person could possibly know it all. Maybe they'll come close with artificial intelligence. However, nothing replaces the presence and energy of human interaction. Either way, when it comes to our health, we are not meant to operate alone as individuals.

For now, we rely on medical specialists to know the intimate details of unique body parts. This can be extremely helpful, and we must appreciate the expertise they bring to the table. Still, it is possible for this piecemeal approach to fail to solve our medical mystery.

MEDICAL SILOS

Maybe you already see a gastroenterologist for your gut, a rheumatologist for your joint pain, an endocrinologist for your thyroid, and a psychologist for your anxiety and depression. Each one has their theory on why you don't feel like yourself. But none is helping you see the whole picture. Medical specialists look at things in silos. Their job is to focus on the one body part they know all about. This can be a very good thing. The trouble with this is that when they refer you to another specialist, the overall understanding of the system as a whole is scattered like dandelion fluff in the wind. We are not silos of body parts. We are whole humans. We have a physical, emotional, cognitive, and spiritual aspect to our being. We are knit together in special ways that make each of us unique.

I remember having some troubles with extreme fatigue. I'd hit a brick wall at three in the afternoon, and my brain would stop functioning. It was like my mind packed up for the day and said, "*That's it. I'm outta here.*" I needed some outside help. I wasn't feeling like myself at all. I'd wake up in the night with pains in my gut, only relieved by taking magnesium or having a small snack. My sense of taste was off. I could barely eat anything without reacting to it. My nervous system was so sensitive even the caffeine in a decaf tea was too much for me. My tendons and my joints were wound tighter than I emotionally felt.

The family physician told me it was perimenopause, the psychiatrist told me it was stress, the endocrinologist finally agreed to adjust my thyroid medication, and my naturopathic doctor told me it was my adrenals. No one was able to tell me why things were happening the way they were, and it was up to me to figure out how to pull myself back together: I had to be my own doctor. Was it helpful to have the insights and testing from all the other physicians? Absolutely. However, I have found that throughout the journey to understand my health woes, it has generally been left to me to figure out how I am knit together. That's what drove me into this line of work. I don't expect everyone to want to get to the same level of detail. I'm not a mechanic, so I like to drive my car without knowing what makes it work. But I do like to know what indicators to watch for so I know when it is time to change my oil, fix my brakes, or get new tires. The intention of this chapter is to show you some health indicators to watch.

DIG INTO DIGESTION

"If someone wishes for good health, one must first ask oneself if he is ready to do away with the reasons for his illness. Only then is it possible to help him."

—HIPPOCRATES

As we learned, the microbiome exists beyond the gut. When the gut lining gets compromised, things that should remain in the gut can travel everywhere.

It's true. Alterations in the gut microbiome (dysbiosis) can lead to serious health complications such as nonalcoholic fatty liver disease, nonalcoholic steatohepatitis, inflammatory bowel disease, depression, fibromyalgia, cardiovascular disease, rheumatoid arthritis, eczema, psoriasis, diabetes mellitus, obesity, and cancer. We need to follow the trail of breadcrumbs. Boy, that saying sure carries more weight than intended. Our inability to properly digest gluten is a major factor in many inflammatory diseases.

Set yourself free from the labels you have been given. Begin with fresh eyes and ears. Some things can't be seen or heard. They are purely sensations in the body. This is where your "gut sense" or intuition may come into play.

ORAL HEALTH

Picture a big, juicy yellow lemon. Now visualize holding on to that lemon and then putting it on a cutting board and slicing into it. Take a quarter of it and slice that so you have an eighth of a lemon. Now imagine putting that lemon up to your lips. Squeeze the tangy juice into your mouth. Pucker power. Is your mouth watering at even the thought of it? Strangely enough, mine does! Your mouth is the beginning of the digestive microbiome. Did you know digestion begins before the food is put into your mouth? Think of food, and your mouth can water.

We are wired to associate finding food with safety. It's a natural survival mechanism built into our genes. What we see, smell, feel, and think about happen in advance of what we taste, let alone swallow. Recall the last time you did the sniff test of something in the fridge. I'll bet you looked at it first, then sniffed it. If the food passed both those tests, then you may have decided it was safe to eat. The mouth is the first point of digestive contact. If a piece of food is really bitter, it's likely not good for us to eat a lot of it. We spit it out. Now, people have different levels of receptor sensitivity to bitter foods. If you are like me, you don't mind bitter things at all. Bitter and sour things are good for your digestion. They stimulate the digestive juices not just in the mouth but in the entire digestive tract. This is why some like to take a cup of hot lemon water early in the day to get things moving. It's a good alternative to coffee.

A dry mouth will impede digestion, promote bacterial overgrowth in the mouth, and reduce your ability to taste and enjoy food. The dryness may not be just in your mouth but the whole digestive tract. If you have a dry colon, this will contribute to dry stool that is difficult to pass and can cause constipation. There are some medications such as nonprescription drugs for allergies and colds, high blood pressure, overactive bladder, and mental health issues that contribute to dry mouth. This makes sense because the goal of those drugs is to dry up some part of your body. Dry mouth is more than being thirsty. If you do not make enough saliva, it is not only uncomfortable but can also lead to digestive issues.

THE INSIDE OF THE MOUTH

What is that blistery bubble inside my cheek? I didn't bite it, although I did just finish my lunch. When I eat too many tomatoes or tart apples, I get mouth cankers. Some people have oral food allergies, most often to tree fruits or citrus fruits. It makes me wonder how the rest of the mucus membranes along the digestive tract might react. Are there sores in my lower intestines, too? Sometimes with or instead of mouth sores, I get tummy aches or constipation when I eat too many tomatoes.

Mouth cankers (aphthous ulcers) can occur with consumption of coffee, chocolate, eggs, cheese, or spicy and acidic foods. They can also come from sodium laurel sulfate in toothpaste or mouthwash, or a deficiency in zinc, B12, folate, or iron.

Sharp pains and burning in the mouth indicate nerve involvement. This can be stress-related as the vagal nerve intricately winds along this path and down to the digestive tract. We will talk about the vagal nerve and stress later in the book. Infection and injury can trigger nerve pain. Do you have mouth pain? What does it feel like? Where exactly does it hurt?

THE GUMS

Receding gum lines can be a point of entry for bacterial infection. Bacteria found in the joints of those with rheumatoid arthritis (RA)[40] are also found in the mouth of those with periodontal disease. DMARDs (disease-modifying antirheumatic drugs) such as methotrexate, sulfasalazine, leflunomide, and hydroxychloroquine show partial restoration of the gut microbiome through immune suppression and anti-inflammatory actions.[41]

When you brush or floss your teeth, is there blood in the sink when you spit? This is a good indication of gum disease.

THE TEETH

Slow down! You just inhaled your dinner. Did you even chew? Eating fast or on the run is not good for digestion.

It is important to have healthy teeth. Their purpose is to chew your food. If you don't chew your food properly, it makes it diffi-

---

40 Mayes, M. D. (1999). Epidemiologic studies of environmental agents and systemic autoimmune diseases. *Environmental Health Perspectives, 107*(Suppl 5), 743–748. https://doi.org/10.1289/ehp.9910785743

41 Bodkhe, R., Balakrishnan, B., & Taneja, V. (2019). The role of microbiome in rheumatoid arthritis treatment. *Therapeutic Advances in Musculoskeletal Disease, 11*, 1759720X19844632. https://doi.org/10.1177/1759720X19844632

cult for the rest of the digestive tract to break it down. Undigested food can be a factor in diarrhea and constipation. Discolored teeth or poor development of enamel can be related to sensitivity to gluten.

UPPER DIGESTIVE HEALTH (ESOPHAGUS, STOMACH, SMALL INTESTINE)

When we can't swallow something, or contents of the stomach rise up from the stomach, push past the lower esophageal sphincter and into the esophagus, we feel pressure, burning, and discomfort. This includes emotional events that are "difficult to swallow."

Food sensitivities are another cause of heartburn. Peppermint, spicy things, chocolate, caffeine, citrus (lemons, limes, grapefruit, oranges), peppers, and alcohol can all be irritants of the sphincter between the esophagus and stomach. When the sphincter gets irritated, it doesn't stay closed. Picture a door with a faulty hinge: when a big breeze comes, the door swings wide open and lets in the cat. In this case, stomach acid and undigested foods comes back up into the esophagus and claw at the tissue.

The stomach is meant to have an acidic environment. It kills invaders, triggers intrinsic factor release so you can absorb vitamin B12, and begins the physical breakdown of proteins. Changes in the stomach's acidic environment send messages that stimulate the pancreas to release digestive enzymes that help the fats (lipases), carbohydrates (amylases), and proteins (proteases) break down.

An overgrowth in bacteria (*Helicobacter pylori*, aka *H. pylori*) in the small intestine or in the stomach can be the root cause of gas, pain, burping, bloating, and belching. Lovely little critter, isn't it? Told you not all of what's going on is your fault! This crafty bug likes to create a very alkaline or basic environment in the stomach.[42]

If there is an overgrowth of H. pylori, it may impact more than your digestion. An imbalance can also lead to chronic inflammation body-wide. This contributes to skin and heart diseases, obesity, anemia, insulin resistance, and nonalcoholic fatty liver disease (NAFLD). If you have it, you are not alone! About half the adults in the world have H. pylori. Most have no symptoms. About 10–15 percent of those infected develop chronic inflammation leading to atrophic gastritis, peptic ulcer, and stomach cancer.[43] Breath tests, blood tests, and stool tests are all available to find out if you have it. There are several related conditions, and treating it with a hot water mushroom extract of lion's mane (Hericium erinaceus) in addition to a gut reset protocol for six to eight weeks will help resolve the symptoms, which include:[44]

· alopecia (balding/hair loss)
· chronic urticaria
· rosacea
· psoriasis

42 Bravo, D., Hoare, A., Soto, C., Valenzuela, M. A., & Quest, A. F. (2018). Helicobacter pylori in human health and disease: Mechanisms for local gastric and systemic effects. World Journal of Gastroenterology, 24(28), 3071–3089. https://doi.org/10.3748/wjg.v24.i28.3071

43 Chattopadhyay, S., Patra, R., Chatterjee, R., De, R., Alam, J., Ramamurthy, T., Chowdhury, A., Nair, G. B., Berg, D. E., & Mukhopadhyay, A. K. (2012). Distinct repeat motifs at the C-terminal region of CagA of Helicobacter pylori strains isolated from diseased patients and asymptomatic individuals in West Bengal, India. Gut Pathogens, 4(1), 4. https://doi.org/10.1186/1757-4749-4-4

44 Campuzano-Maya, G. (2011). Cure of alopecia areata after eradication of Helicobacter pylori: A new association? World Journal of Gastroenterology, 17(26), 3165–3170. https://doi.org/10.3748/wjg.v17.i26.3165

- Schönlein-Henoch purpura
- Behçet's disease
- prurigo nodularis
- chronic cutaneous pruritus
- progressive systemic sclerosis
- Sjögren's syndrome
- Sweet's syndrome

H. pylori isn't all bad. When introduced into a body that is still young, it may be protective against celiac disease, inflammatory bowel disease, and asthma in children.

On the flip side, sometimes stomach pain can result from too much acid. If you take a lot of nonsteroidal anti-inflammatories (NSAIDs) without food, over time they can erode the gut lining, and ulcers will form. Stomach ulcers are very painful sores in the mucosal membrane, and the acid they release will really burn— like alcohol on an open wound.

So how do you identify the cause of your pain? Medical imaging with a scope might help. But I would say low stomach acid is much more common than high, especially if there is not much cause for ulcers to build (you don't have a history of long-term, frequent use of NSAIDs). Still, the prescription of proton-pump inhibitors, which reduce acid in your stomach, is widespread and not always necessary because it is assumed too much acid is the problem, but often it is not.

Consider someone with bad breath and heartburn. They may also complain about numbness or tingling in their hands and feet, muscle cramps, dizziness, trouble remembering things, fatigue, and depression. There is a risk of B12 depletion when an over-growth of *H. pylori* is reducing the stomach acid to make itself a cozy living environment. Symptoms of B12 deficiency are like those of old age. If you have heartburn and feel older than you are, look into it. Not all B12 deficiencies are easily recognizable or diagnosed. Even people whose blood work reveals normal B12 levels can present with deficiency symptoms.

LIVER HEALTH

Stephanie, 32, came to see me as a new patient. Her medical doctor had diagnosed her with nonalcoholic fatty liver disease (NAFLD) two weeks prior. She sought help with diet and supplements. She was overweight and didn't care much for exercise but was now highly motivated to change. Her liver enzymes were elevated, and ultrasound results confirmed her diagnosis. She starts immediately on a diet of greens, a little bit of olive oil and vinegar, protein (beef, chicken, fish, or vegan protein powder), and one cup of blueberries per day. That's it. No other food. Exercise is at least thirty minutes a day to move her body: walking and a weight-lifting routine at home. I give Stephanie a liver-support tincture with *Silymarin*, *Scutelaria baclensis*, *White atractylodes*, *Bupluerum*, and *Gentian lutea*. One teaspoon on rising, wait fifteen minutes before food. One activated B complex with breakfast, plus 1,000 mg vitamin C and 1,000 IU vitamin D. Thorne Mediclear vegan protein powder, one scoop in smoothie for breakfast. Magnesium bisglycinate 400 mg before bed.

Four months later, Stephanie has lost twenty pounds, her liver enzymes are back to normal, and ultrasound confirms she has reversed her NAFLD. Her maintenance diet is paleolithic: no grains, lots of lean protein and greens, and only one fruit a day (blueberries, an apple, or half a grapefruit). Supplements now are a mixed probiotic 11 billion per day once daily with food, fish oil, 1,000 IU vitamin D, 1,000 mg vitamin C, one capsule activated B complex, and 400 mg magnesium before bed.

What had happened to Stephanie? She didn't drink much alcohol. How did she end up with liver disease?

Overindulgence in carbohydrates and resulting insulin resistance can lead to a fatty liver. When you eat, energy is stored in the muscles for later use. When those stores are full, the liver will take some of the excess. Then the fat stores build up. In childhood, a fatty liver can be caused by a variety of disorders, including those related to problems with copper metabolism (e.g., Wilson disease), viral hepatitis, or a variety of autoimmune diseases. It is also a result of higher childhood and early adolescent overindulgence.[45]

Note that NAFLD may progress to steatohepatitis, liver cirrhosis, and even hepatocellular carcinoma. Don't wait—get help before it gets more serious. Stephanie did, and she is now on a much better path.

"Things sweet to taste prove in digestion sour."

—WILLIAM SHAKESPEARE, *RICHARD II*

The liver plays many roles in the body. It has a direct portal

---

45   Anderson, E. L., Howe, L. D., Fraser, A., Macdonald-Wallis, C., Callaway, M. P., Sattar, N., Day, C., Tilling, K., & Lawlor, D. A. (2015). Childhood energy intake is associated with nonalcoholic fatty liver disease in adolescents. *The Journal of Nutrition*, 145(5), 983-989. https://doi.org/10.3945/jn.114.208397

(hepatoportal vein) from the gastrointestinal tract. When the microbiome is disturbed, the gut lining cells are damaged (leaky gut), and bad bacteria and their toxins from the gut harm the liver.[46] If they don't receive treatment, those with celiac disease are eight times more likely to die of liver cirrhosis.[47] Abnormal liver blood tests may be the only clue to celiac disease.

GALLBLADDER HEALTH

Like a major intersection, the gallbladder, pancreas, stomach, and liver all come to a crossroads with their ducts. Sometimes the bile here gets thick and goopy. Bile is 95 percent water, and the remaining 5 percent is cholesterol, bile salts, proteins, steroids, enzymes, vitamins, and toxins (heavy metals, xenoestrogens, drug-breakdown products). With all that "stuff," no wonder it can form a sludge, which can block the ducts or dry to make stones in the gallbladder. Pain in the right shoulder blade is commonly attributed to stones moving against the walls of the gallbladder or ducts.

There's a little-known link between gallstones and celiac disease. Early detection of celiac disease could save you from gallbladder surgery. Cholesystokinin (CCK) is normally released in the small intestine in response to a fatty meal. But if the small intestine is damaged from gluten or other factors, then the cells that release the CCK may be unresponsive. They can't do their job. CCK is needed to trigger the gallbladder to release its bile. If bile is not

46 Konturek, P. C., Harsch, I. A., Konturek, K., Schink, M., Konturek, T., Neurath, M. F., & Zopf, Y. (2018). Gut-liver axis: How do gut bacteria influence the liver? *Medical Sciences, 6*(3), 79. https://doi.org/10.3390/medsci6030079

47 Rubio-Tapia, A., & Murray, J. A. (2007). The liver in celiac disease. *Hepatology, 46*(5), 1650–1658. https://doi.org/10.1002/hep.21949

released, it hangs around and gets sludgy (which increases risk of gallstones). Without proper bile, the fat in the meal will be poorly digested. In those with inflammatory bowel disease, this could be one reason for diarrhea after eating.[48]

PANCREAS

We often think of the pancreas when it comes to diabetes, blood sugar regulation, and insulin control.

The pancreas can be evaluated through blood tests that check levels of its enzymes, amylase, and lipase. Enzymes are chemical scissors that break food down into smaller, more absorbable pieces. High levels of these enzymes indicate pancreatic inflammation (pancreatitis). About 20 percent of those who suffer from celiac disease also have pancreatic issues.[49] These can result from genetic factors or from the body's failure to absorb enough proteins for the pancreas to function.

You'll notice I mention celiac disease quite often. Gluten or wheat-related intolerances may affect the gut's connection to the health of the rest of your body. It is a common offender that should not go without consideration. That said, it's not the cause of everything. And sticking to a gluten-free diet isn't always enough.

---

48 Wang, H. H., Liu, M., Li, X., Portincasa, P., & Wang, D. Q. (2017). Impaired intestinal cholecystokinin secretion, a fascinating but overlooked link between coeliac disease and cholesterol gallstone disease. *European Journal of Clinical Investigation, 47*(4), 328–333. https://doi.org/10.1111/eci.12734

49 Carroccio, A., Iacono, G., Montalto, G., Cavataio, F., Di Marco, C., Balsamo, V., & Notarbartolo, A. (1991). Exocrine pancreatic function in children with coeliac disease before and after a gluten free diet. *Gut, 32*(7), 796–799. https://doi.org/10.1136/gut.32.7.796

SMALL INTESTINE

Small intestinal bacterial overgrowth (SIBO) is a common condition of the gut.

SIBO can result from inflammation, stagnant food, or lazy valves.

What's going on with SIBO? The microbes that should stay in the large intestine start making it up to the small intestine. When they start to work on food that is not broken down enough, it causes gas, pain, bloating, and fatigue. This happens because of fermentation. When carbohydrates ferment rather than digest, hydrogen and methane can be produced in measurable quantities. Food stagnates with poor gut motility (movement of food along the channel) as in hypothyroid, because the food stays around longer and has more opportunity to ferment.

Symptoms related to SIBO are nausea, flatulence, bad breath, diarrhea, constipation, alternating diarrhea and constipation (IBS), leaky gut syndrome, chronic fatigue syndrome, acid reflux, rosacea (red, rough patches on the face), achy muscles and joints, and heartburn.

If you have celiac or Crohn's disease, the small intestine is absolutely at risk. In people with celiac disease, the immune system mistakes gluten for an invader and builds resistance to it. The trouble is that gluten proteins look a lot like the proteins in the lining of the small intestine. So over time, the lining gets destroyed because the body thinks the proteins in it are bad guys. It's like burning a healthy forest to the ground. But the proteins in the lining also look a lot like muscle layers in other parts of the body. This is why those with fibromyalgia, polymyalgia, cerebellar ataxia, or multiple sclerosis do so much better on a gluten-free diet. It's called molecular mimicry. Think about a doppelganger—a being that looks so much like another it could be mistaken for it.

Don't discount the possibility that you have celiac disease based on the results of your antibody tests—up to 7 percent of people with celiac disease test negative. If this is you and you still suspect you have celiac and are still eating gluten, press on to get the small intestine (duodenal) biopsy.[50] Or consider other wheat-related protein tests such as the Cyrex Array 3x or Wheat Zoomer or HLA-DQ2 or HLA-DQ8 genetic test. (More on tests in chapter 5.)

Normally, the immune defence would only trigger a reaction against really bad guys, but in people with Crohn's disease, there are fights among commonly helpful microbes. A variety of factors can stir the pot and cause these fights. An overgrowth of bacterium *Ruminococcus gnavus* is associated with both Crohn's disease and systemic lupus erythematosus.[51] Keep in mind, additional factors such as genetics, immune system problems, and environmental factors also contribute to the onset of any chronic disease (including Crohn's, SLE, and celiac disease).

Lazy valves often occur as a result of inflammation. If the ileocecal (IC) valve between the small intestine and large intestine gets irritated, it doesn't close properly. Contents of the large intestine

---

50 Arasaradnam, R. P., Brown, S., Forbes, A., Fox, M. R., Hungin, P., Kelman, L., Major, G., O'Connor, M., Sanders, D. S., Sinha, R., Smith, S. C., Thomas, P., & Walters, J. (2018). Guidelines for the investigation of chronic diarrhoea in adults: British Society of Gastroenterology, 3rd edition. *Gut, 67*(8), 1380–1399. https://doi.org/10.1136/gutjnl-2017-315909

51 Kim, J. W., Kwok, S. K., Choe, J. Y., & Park, S. H. (2019). Recent advances in our understanding of the link between the intestinal microbiota and systemic lupus erythematosus. *International Journal of Molecular Sciences, 20*(19), 4871. https://doi.org/10.3390/ijms20194871

infect the small intestine. This can cause a deep achy pain to the right of your navel and down a little.

Jane's Gut Pain Vanishes

I once had a patient, Jane, who came in because she had this ache in her tummy for two years. I say once, because I saw her once and then never again. For two years, no conventional doctor could help Jane with this constant gnawing pain. Appendicitis ruled out, I was up for the challenge. When I had my hands on her abdomen, I could feel the tension around the ileocecal valve: just to the right of and a little lower than her navel. With a hands-on adjustment, I was able to close the valve for her. She never returned for her follow-up appointment. Initially, I was a bit worried the treatment had offended her. Poking in the belly is not all that fun, and the spot was pretty tender. So I called her on the phone to check in. *"Jane, is everything all right? How was your experience after your initial appointment?"* Jane said, *"Yes, sorry, I didn't let you know. After you did that adjustment, my pain was gone before I left your office that day. I have never felt it again, and I am doing great."*

Gut inflammation from fungal overgrowth, leaky IC valve, food sensitivities, bacteria overgrowth, viral infections, and other environmental toxins irritate and inflame the lining of the gastrointestinal tract. Then you get leaky gut. Things that should stay in the gut get into the bloodstream. This means toxins, and even chunks of food that would normally stay in the gut to get broken down into itty-bitty pieces, escape. Fungal colonies set up satellite offices everywhere. Just like fungi found on the forest floor, which spread their communication networks out over many square miles,[52] fungi can easily spread throughout the entire body. Their unusual presence in the bloodstream puts the immune system on high alert because it considers them an invader.

When the immune system is activated, there is inflammation. Inflammation can trigger pain and disease in different parts of the body. It can be a factor in depression, headaches, joint pain, and skin issues. Long-term increased inflammation contributes to insulin resistance, which is a stepping stone to obesity and type 2 diabetes.[53] All this from things going wrong in the small intestine.

You smelled the food, tasted the food, chewed the food (hopefully), and swallowed the food. The subsequent digestive steps are largely beyond your influence. Once you put the food down there, you just hope for the best. The body takes over. Generally, you don't pay much attention to a well-functioning gut. As with a grown child who's moved out of the house, you only hear from it when something is wrong.

No news is generally good news, we say at our house. I suppose, however, since you are reading this book, you've recently gotten a phone call from your gut. It could be the microbes kicking up a fuss. The microbiome is like a village of children we carry around inside of us.

If you are quiet enough in your own body, you'll know what's up with it. Just like if you know your children well enough to watch

---

52 Wohlleben, P. (2016). *The hidden life of trees*. Greystone Books.

53 Scheithauer, T. P., Dallinga-Thie, G. M., de Vos, W. M., Nieuwdorp, M., & van Raalte, D. H. (2016). Causality of small and large intestinal microbiota in weight regulation and insulin resistance. *Molecular Metabolism*, 5(9), 759–770. https://doi.org/10.1016/j.molmet.2016.06.002

their behaviour and know when the sky is about to fall in. But when you don't have all of the information, it can be tough to come to a conclusion. You need the *whole* truth.

LOWER INTESTINAL TRACT (APPENDIX, LARGE INTESTINE, RECTUM, AND ANUS)

Appendix

The appendix is the sacred jewel queen of the microbiome. When things such as stress, diet, infection, or antibiotics upset the microbiome, the appendix restores balance to your digestive kingdom. From its sacred stores, it provides you with your own personal probiotic infusion.[54] Boy, I could use a healthy inoculation from my appendix right about now. How about you?

The appendix, however, may be to blame when it comes to ulcerative colitis. Colitis is an inflammatory bowel disease that makes your immune system attack its own microbiome. The main symptoms are blood and mucous in diarrhea. Removal of the appendix in those suffering from colitis can be one way to remission.[55]

Large Intestine

The large intestine starts at the lower right corner of your belly area, goes up to your rib cage, follows the border of the rib cage across, then goes down the left side of your belly. It takes a bit of a turn before it meets the exit at the bum, or anus. Up to 95 per-

---

54 Vitetta, L., Chen, J., & Clarke, S. (2019). The vermiform appendix: An immunological organ sustaining a microbiome inoculum. *Clinical Science, 133*(1), 1–8. https://doi.org/10.1042/CS20180956

55 Sahami, S., Kooij, I. A., Meijer, S. L., van den Brink, G. R., Buskens, C. J., & te Velde, A. A. (2016). The link between the appendix and ulcerative colitis: Clinical relevance and potential immunological mechanisms. *The American Journal of Gastroenterology, 111*(2), 163–169. https://doi.org/10.1038/ajg.2015.301

cent of the bacteria in the gut microbiome are located in the large intestine. The large intestine continues to digest what the small intestine could not: walls of plant cells, cellulose, hemicelluloses, pectin, and resistant starch.[56]

Microbial fermentation of carbohydrates and proteins occurs in the large intestine. Fermentation makes short-chain fatty acids (SCFAs). We don't want fermentation in the small intestine, but we do want it in the large intestine. We need the products of fermentation (SCFAs) in the large intestine to feed the cells lining the gut, regulate immune function, and reduce inflammation.

Different microbes produce different types of SCFAs. The SCFA balance is incredibly important. When the microbiome in the large intestine changes, so does the balance of SCFAs. This can contribute to how the gut signals the feeling of fullness to the brain (satiety), fat, and glucose metabolism.[57] Imbalances in SCFAs also affect how proteins fold in the brain, a leading factor in Alzheimer's disease.[58]

What can go wrong in the large intestine? Colitis, polyps, cancer, diverticula.

As mentioned above, colitis is marked by a bloody loose stool. People with colitis have a microbe war going on in their colon,

---

56 Bäckhed, F., Ley, R. E., Sonnenburg, J. L., Peterson, D. A., & Gordon, J. I. (2005). Host-bacterial mutualism in the human intestine. *Science, 307*(5717), 1915-1920. https://doi.org/10.1126/science.1104816

57 Zhou, D., & Fan, J. G. (2019). Microbial metabolites in non-alcoholic fatty liver disease. *World Journal of Gastroenterology, 25*(17), 2019-2028. https://doi.org/10.3748/wjg.v25.i17.2019

58 Marizzoni, M., Cattaneo, A., Mirabelli, P., Festari, C., Lopizzo, N., Nicolosi, V., Mombelli, E., Mazzelli, M., Luongo, D., Naviglio, D., Coppola, L., Salvatore, M., & Frisoni, G. B. (2020). Short-chain fatty acids and lipopolysaccharide as mediators between gut dysbiosis and amyloid pathology in Alzheimer's disease. *Journal of Alzheimer's Disease, 78*(2), 683-697. https://doi.org/10.3233/JAD-200306

where the immune system begins to target a normally helpful part of the gut microbiome. This can cause tenderness and irritation in the lining of the large intestine.

There are different types of microbes down here, and this is where fibre is super important in the diet. You need soluble, or soft, fibre to attract water into the stool so it is soft. You need bulky insoluble fibre to provide "roughage" to move the stool through, like a corn broom sweeping it away.

Talk about sweeping. The muscles around the large and small intestine are bidirectional. Some go around like elastic bands, and some go lengthwise down the tube. When these muscles contract, it helps move the food along the processing line. When you are stressed, it affects your nervous system, which can mess up the firing of these gut motility muscles. This can lead to either diarrhea or constipation.

Constipation can occur for many different reasons. One is motility. As mentioned earlier, medications such as opioids and pain meds can really bring the processing line to a halt. When you strain to excrete, that's not good either. This can also happen in hypothyroidism—when basically everything in the body slows down. If the colon is too dry, dehydration and lack of dietary fibre can be factors.

In the past, humans took in about 28 g of fibre a day. In modern times, fibre intake is more like 2–4 g for most standard American diets. No wonder it is nicknamed the SAD diet. It makes the body very sad. We will talk more about what to eat in chapter 4. How does what goes on in the large intestine affect the rest of the body? Well, when waste sticks around too long, as during constipation, things start getting reabsorbed that are really meant to be excreted. In it goes, loading up your toxic bucket. And the lining of the large intestine can get sore.

Diverticulitis

Straining when you go to the bathroom? All that pressure has to go somewhere, so you end up with hemorrhoids, which are weak veins bursting out, or diverticula, which are out pouches of tissue in the colon wall. Material can get stuck in the diverticula and cause inflammation (diverticulitis). This painful condition usually happens in the lower left side of the belly. A great tincture made of plant medicines (*Chelidonium majus*, *Dioscorea villosa*, *Hydrastis canendensis*, *Commiphora myrrh*) often serves to treat diverticulitis. Some also find eliminating seeds, fruits with seeds (think strawberries, raspberries, sesame), and nuts can help.

Polyps

Clumps of cells tend to form in the colon when a person doesn't eat enough vegetables on a regular basis. Over time, the clumps build into a polyp. Over time, the polyp can become cancerous. How does this happen? A low intake of fibre (less than 15 g per day) leads to less variety of microbes in the gut, which means fewer SCFAs. SCFAs help reduce the chance of inflammation and polyp formation.[59] Low levels of one particular SCFA, butyrate, are

---

59   Zeng, H., Umar, S., Rust, B., Lazarova, D., & Bordonaro, M. (2019). Secondary bile acids and short chain fatty acids in the colon: A focus on colonic microbiome, cell proliferation, inflammation, and cancer. *International Journal of Molecular Sciences*, 20(5), 1214. https://doi.org/10.3390/ijms20051214

linked to increased risk of colitis[60] and colon cancer.[61] Without enough butyrate, the body uses secondary bile acids to regenerate the gut lining. These acids are very inflammatory. If you don't have diverticulitis, this is a very good reason to eat nuts, seeds, a little fruit, and vegetables! See how foods can both harm and heal? Depends on the dose and depends on the circumstances.

Rectum and Anus

Rectal fissures, fistulas, and hemorrhoids are a result of weak vein walls and straining to relieve stool. You may notice streaks of red on the toilet paper when you wipe, a burning sensation as stool exits, or pain in the area. Trauma can be internal or external. Many people with colitis also suffer from fissures or fistulas. Many people with varicose veins on the legs also experience hemorrhoids. Both are due to a similar underlying mechanism. To help heal this area, I've prescribed capsules with *Boswellia serata* or with *Aesculus hippocastanum*, a homeopathic such as Arsenicum album 30 CH or Calc Sulph 30 K, and a topical homeopathic ointment by Unda called Proctasan.

Dark stool like coffee grounds is more concerning because it means there is bleeding farther up the gastrointestinal tract. Either way, these things should be recorded and discussed with your medical provider.

Itchy bum? Especially at night? You could have a parasitic

---

60 Ganapathy, V., Thangaraju, M., Prasad, P. D., Martin, P. M., & Singh, N. (2013). Transporters and receptors for short-chain fatty acids as the molecular link between colonic bacteria and the host. *Current Opinion in Pharmacology*, 13(6), 869–874. https://doi.org/10.1016/j.coph.2013.08.006

61 Gonçalves, P., & Martel, F. (2013). Butyrate and colorectal cancer: The role of butyrate transport. *Current Drug Metabolism*, 14(9), 994–1008. https://doi.org/10.2174/1389200211314090006

infection, or pinworm, or *Candida* overgrowth. Time for some comprehensive stool analysis.

NERVOUS SYSTEM

The organs of digestion, as discussed above, are controlled by a mesh of nerves that govern the gastrointestinal tract (known as the enteric nervous system) and the central nervous system, which includes your brain and spinal tract.

The relation between the microbiome and the nervous system is now referred to as the gut-brain axis. The microbes in the gut communicate with the brain.[62] Your microbiome is a communication network that acts within the nervous, hormone, and endocrine systems. This makes it an integral part of the gut-brain axis and why your mood can be a reflection of, or reaction to, what's going on in your gut. The microbiome monitors gut function and integrates the emotional and rational centres of the brain.[63]

Gut bacteria can directly stimulate the nervous system of the gut (the enteric nervous system), which, in turn, triggers the vagus nerve to send messages to the brain. From the microbiome, *Lactobacillus* and *Bifidobacterium* use the vagus nerve for

62   Ma, Q., Xing, C., Long, W., Wang, H. Y., Liu, Q., & Wang, R. F. (2019). Impact of microbiota on central nervous system and neurological diseases: The gut-brain axis. *Journal of Neuroinflammation, 16*(1), 53. https://doi.org/10.1186/s12974-019-1434-3

63   Carabotti, M., Scirocco, A., Maselli, M. A., & Severi, C. (2015). The gut-brain axis: Interactions between enteric microbiota, central and enteric nervous systems. *Annals of Gastroenterology, 28*(2), 203–209.

bidirectional communication between the gut and the brain.[64] In one laboratory example, *Bifidobacterium* specifically helps calm colitis-related anxiety. If the vagus connection is severed, the anxiety behavior returns.[65]

Your gut microbes affect your feelings and make you think. Literally. The short-chain fatty acids (SCFAs) made in the lower intestine of the gut also communicate directly to the sympathetic (fight or flight) nervous system, stimulate gut serotonin release, and influence memory and learning.[66]

Immune response against gluten and dairy proteins can cross-react to cells in the cerebellum and myelin sheath. That means if you are sensitive to dairy and wheat, you may have more than irritable bowel syndrome to worry about. The cerebellum controls balance, and the myelin sheath insulates nerve fibres so they can send messages quickly. Breakdown of the myelin sheath is a frequent observation in multiple sclerosis.

Immune response against gluten and dairy proteins can also cross-react to an enzyme involved in the production of GABA. GABA (gamma-aminobutyric acid) weakens or slows down nervous system transmission (calms an excited nervous system)

64 Bravo, J. A., Forsythe, P., Chew, M. V., Escaravage, E., Savignac, H. M., Dinan, T. G., Bienenstock, J., & Cryan, J. F. (2011). Ingestion of *Lactobacillus* strain regulates emotional behavior and central GABA receptor expression in a mouse via the vagus nerve. *Proceedings of the National Academy of Sciences of the United States of America*, *108*(38), 16050-16055. https://doi.org/10.1073/pnas.1102999108

65 Bercik, P., Park, A. J., Sinclair, D., Khoshdel, A., Lu, J., Huang, X., Deng, Y., Blennerhassett, P. A., Fahnestock, M., Moine, D., Berger, B., Huizinga, J. D., Kunze, W., McLean, P. G., Bergonzelli, G. E., Collins, S. M., & Verdu, E. F. (2011). The anxiolytic effect of *Bifidobacterium longum* NCC3001 involves vagal pathways for gut-brain communication. *Neurogastroenterology and Motility*, *23*(12), 1132-1139. https://doi.org/10.1111/j.1365-2982.2011.01796.x

66 Carabotti, M., Scirocco, A., Maselli, M. A., & Severi, C. (2015). The gut-brain axis: Interactions between enteric microbiota, central and enteric nervous systems. *Annals of Gastroenterology*, *28*(2), 203-209.

and relaxes muscle tone. Without it, we feel anxious. Low levels of *Lactobacillus rhamnosus* can impact GABA production, too. Wheat and dairy sensitivity and microbiome imbalance all contribute to depression and anxiety.[67]

You might feel a little bored because not everything in this chapter pertains to you. Allow it. Take a moment to notice how your body feels in this moment. Is it tight and contracted or soft and expansive? Be very thankful not all this stuff affects you. Often, patients come to me with numerous chronic health issues, having never once considered the factor of gut health. You're very fortunate if you can catch things early or recognize the root causes of your problems.

Take some time to yourself and appreciate the difference a balanced microbiome and healthy gut lining can make! Maybe you know someone who also needs to learn this difference.

Next, find some music that resonates with your soul and listen with your whole body. Absorb its vibrations. Maybe even move your body to it in some creative way. When you come back, you'll realize you're already on your way to better health. As you will learn in the next chapter, it is important to make changes one bite at a time.

---

67   Dhakal, R., Bajpai, V. K., & Baek, K. H. (2012). Production of GABA (γ-aminobutyric acid) by microorganisms: A review. *Brazilian Journal of Microbiology, 43*(4), 1230–1241. https://doi.org/10.1590/S1517-83822012000400001

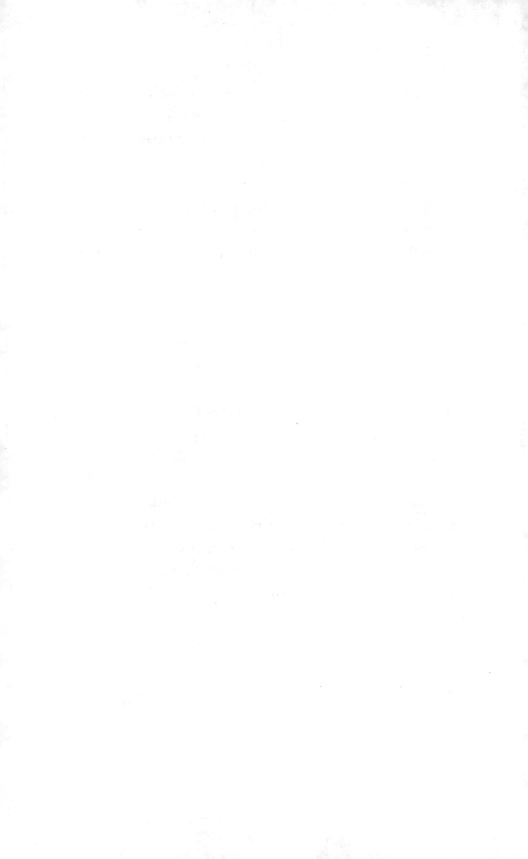

ONE BITE AT A TIME

Here's what you'll learn in this chapter:

- How to track your food and how you feel
- An overview of popular "diets"
- Building blocks of healthy food choices
- There's no one right diet for everyone, and dietary needs change to suit your current health status or goals.

"Our food should be our medicine and our medicine should be our food."

—HIPPOCRATES

Food is medicine. Love is, too. I believe we can actually bake love into our food. It's the secret ingredient!

We have a very interesting relationship with food. What is food to you? Necessity? Convenience? Flavour? Enjoyment? Pain?

You don't need to hide anything. I won't judge you. We want to find a style of eating that helps you achieve your current goal. We might change it up later. Don't even call it a diet. Tell me I am going on a diet and all I want to do is eat! Don't deprive me! But give me a good reason to eat or not eat something, and I can stick to it. Easy. Even if it makes me grumpy for a while.

This is not about will power. It is about finding what your body needs that it isn't getting. Think of it like a kid who wants to eat only chocolate chip cookies all the time. If this were your child, would you allow it? My girlfriend in high school got this fabulous job at the most coveted ice-cream parlour in town. I'm talking creamy, dreamy stuff. They got to eat as much ice cream as they wanted. I couldn't imagine it! Then she explained, "*You eat and eat and eat and then you get sick of it. You don't even want a bite. You've just put yourself out of the ice-cream eating business.*" The same can happen when you recognize the pain a certain food causes. Eat enough of it, and you just might remember what it does to you. Unless you have food amnesia. Some do. They'll eat something they know will bother them and don't care. Or don't recall the anguish they experience after eating it. Until they experience it again. It seems silly, but I have met very intelligent people who continue to put themselves in harm's way.

I gather that if you are reading this book, you are tired of feeling like crap all the time.

On a chart like the diet diary included in the appendix, record what you eat as you eat it. Don't think twice; just keep track. Try to be true to yourself. Also, jot down how you feel. Take note of whichever symptoms bother you. Do this every day for a week. This will help you see patterns in your habits and hang-ups.

DO YOU KNOW WHAT TO EAT?

There are many diets out there said to relieve irritable bowel syndrome or disease. Evidently, there is a diet to "fix" just about anything. Regardless of what a particular diet may set out to achieve, every body still needs its basic nutrient building blocks to sustain life.

You need healthy fats to build cell membranes, insulate your nerve fibres, and construct hormones for good message conduction. Proteins are the building blocks of DNA, RNA, muscle, bone, organs, and neurotransmitters. Carbohydrates provide energy to think, move, and build your body. Who doesn't want that? Finally, you need lots of vegetables to provide the polyphenols, minerals, antioxidants, fibre, flavonoids, and phytosterols that help you eliminate toxins and waste. Did you know vegetables contain over 5,000 compounds (plus, likely, many more that are yet to be discovered)?

Why all the differences in diets? We are each our own unique chemistry experiment. Your microbiome and your genes are unlike anyone else's. They interact with one another and are greatly influenced by what you eat. I'll cover a few common diets; then we will discuss a strategy, rather than a diet, that works.

KETO

High-fat diets are known to increase inflammation, intestinal permeability, and shifts in location of bacterial colonies.[68] However, the results may depend on the type of fat. Sources of what fats are allowed in a keto diet are not clear. You will often see variations of plans that may or may not include saturated fat, such as fatty cuts of meat, processed meats, lard, and butter. Usually, it includes monounsaturated fats such as palm and coconut oil, as well as sources of unsaturated fats, such as nuts, seeds, avocados, plant oils, and oily fish. You'll learn more about how to balance your fats later in this chapter. The keto diet provides less than 50 g of carbohydrate a day, forcing the body to switch from a carbohydrate fuel burner to a fat fuel burner. Traditionally, ketogenic diets are helpful for those suffering from seizures and metabolic concerns. Short-term (three to six months) adherence to a keto diet may help reset your insulin sensitivity and improve your body's ability to burn fat (lose weight).[69] But long-term keto may impair thyroid function. Once the insulin is reset and the weight is lost, it's time to modify your diet.

VEGAN, VEGETARIAN, PESCO-VEGETARIAN

Some people find they digest plant-based foods better. Vegan (no animal products whatsoever) and vegetarian (will eat dairy and eggs but no other animal products) have also been around for ages. The pesco-vegetarian eats the same as the vegetarian plus fish. The pescos have to be careful to rotate their fish sources to

68 Abdul Rahim, M., Chilloux, J., Martinez-Gili, L., Neves, A. L., Myridakis, A., Gooderham, N., & Dumas, M. E. (2019). Diet-induced metabolic changes of the human gut microbiome: Importance of short-chain fatty acids, methylamines and indoles. *Acta Diabetologica*, 56(5), 493–500. https://doi.org/10.1007/s00592-019-01312-x

69 Cabrera-Mulero, A., Tinahones, A., Bandera, B., Moreno-Indias, I., Macías-González, M., & Tinahones, F. J. (2019). Keto microbiota: A powerful contributor to host disease recovery. *Reviews in Endocrine & Metabolic Disorders*, 20(4), 415–425. https://doi.org/10.1007/s11154-019-09518-8

avoid heavy metal contamination from our waterways. All may need to supplement and monitor their iron and B12 levels.

PALEO

The paleolithic diet is one like our ancestors ate millions of years ago. Paleo dieters eat meats (especially organ meats), fish and shellfish, eggs, fruits and vegetables, nuts and seeds, herbs and spices, and starches such as potatoes and sweet potatoes, along with healthy fats. Although not likely in our ancestral diet, full-fat dairy products and legumes are part of some paleo diets. Paleo-autoimmune diet restricts the consumption of one or all of the following: nuts, eggs, grains, beans, legumes, dairy, seeds, nightshades (tomatoes, potatoes, eggplant, and peppers), as well as food chemicals and additives. Chris Kresser's *Paleo Cure* is a great resource.

SPECIFIC CARBOHYDRATE

The specific carbohydrate diet is designed for those with Crohn's, ulcerative colitis, diverticulitis, celiac disease, cystic fibrosis, and chronic diarrhea. The essence of it is to provide very specific carbohydrates, with the goal to heal the gastrointestinal tract. It is an alternative to the high-fibre, low-fat, low-residue, anti-yeast, gluten-free diets often used to relieve inflammatory bowel conditions. It removes certain carbohydrates, especially lactose and sucrose, and any other compound of sugar or carbohydrate. The only carbohydrates allowed are those found in fruits, honey, and specially prepared yogurt (no lactase remains), and a few nuts and vegetables. It is believed that due to an unhealthy shift in microbiome, more complex molecular structures of carbohydrates are unable to break down, subsequently ferment, and cause gas, pain, bloating, and abnormal brain function. It is a very strict diet that, over time, will rebalance the microbiome. Eventually, some foods will be reintroduced. The specific carbohydrate diet is similar to but not the same as the FODMAP diet.

FODMAP

FODMAPs are fermentable oligo-, di-, monosaccharides, and polyols. Not only is that a mouthful, the list of FODMAP foods is long and avoiding them all can make eating a real challenge. That's where a food sensitivity test will help narrow things down for you. Otherwise, you may choose to try the FODMAP-free diet, as a process of elimination for three months, then reintroduce items that don't cause problems one by one. An intolerance to FODMAPs may be a major cause of the diarrhea part of irritable bowel syndrome (IBS).

FODMAPs include five categories of sugars: fructose, fructans, lactose, polyols, and galactans. Levels of FODMAP will vary from food to food. This means you may be sensitive to one sugar but not another, or you may be okay with a small collective amount but must be careful not to overwhelm your system. If the microbiome imbalance is corrected, you may be able to go back to eating FODMAP foods again. This can take up to two years of abstinence. Like you and I can be stubborn at times, so can those microbes in the gut!

Just like those with a lactase enzyme deficiency cannot effectively process milk products, those with large intake of fructose or other FODMAP foods may overwhelm the digestive capacity of the small intestine. In those with sensitivities, the FODMAP passes through the small intestine undigested, then ferments when it reaches the large intestine.

There is more than just lactose, sugar, and gluten sensitivity at play when it comes to FODMAPs. According to Eamonn M. Quigley, MD, director of the Lynda K. and David M. Underwood Center for Digestive Disorders at Houston Methodist Hospital, *"As many as 70%-80% of patients with IBS may benefit, to a certain degree, from the low-FODMAP diet."*[70]

Fructose

Fructose is high in sugary foods such as soft drinks, which often have "high-fructose corn syrup" on the label. It also occurs in white sugar, honey, many fruits (dried ones and fresh ones such as apples, mangoes, pears, and watermelon), and vegetables (sugar snap peas, artichokes, and asparagus).

Fructans

When fructose molecules link together in chains, they form fructans. Fructans are abundant in wheat. They are also found in agave, artichokes, asparagus, leeks, garlic, onions (including spring onions), and rye. Some of these are essential to feed the gut. Many prebiotics include artichokes, asparagus, leeks, garlic, onions, and wheat. If you have an imbalance in your microbiome and thus lack the appropriate enzymes to break down FODMAP foods in the small intestine, you can end up with fermentation of

---

70 Piljac Zegarac, J. (2019, August 23). The low-FODMAP diet for IBS: What you need to know. https://www.medscape.com/viewarticle/917069_print

the fructans in the large intestine. This results in gas, pain, bloat, constipation, and diarrhea. The bloat can be really bad. I've seen some people bloat so much they look pregnant!

Non-celiac wheat sensitivity may be a sensitivity to FODMAPs. It also means that diet drinks and chewing gum might upset your stomach. It also might explain why it's easier to eat wheat in Europe than in North America.

What's the difference between wheat (gluten, gliadin) sensitivity and FODMAP sensitivity? FODMAPs cause gastrointestinal (GI) complaints. Gluten and gliadin proteins, on the other hand, may or may not cause GI complaints, whereas they do cause a lack of well-being in every other part of the body. European wheat is lower in FODMAPs than North American wheat, so if you're sensitive and you eat it, you'll still get an immune response, just not the GI complaints.

Galactins

Galactins are also a FODMAP food. Chickpeas (garbanzo beans), legumes, lentils, pistachio nuts, and cashews top this list.

Methane- and hydrogen-sensitive breath tests available through your naturopathic or functional medicine doctor can help identify the causes and symptoms (gas, pain, bloating, bad breath) of carbohydrate (FODMAP) malabsorption. SIBO (small intestinal bacterial overgrowth) can exacerbate the issue.

Lactose

Lactase enzyme is required to break down the milk sugar lactose. Sixty-eight percent of the world is lactase deficient. This reaches as high as 100 percent in the Han Chinese population. With age, it is natural to loose lactase levels. For those with FODMAP sensitivity to lactose, lactose-free milk products may be tolerable.

Polyols

You might recognize polyols as an ingredient in items labeled sugar-free. Watch for them in gum, mouthwash, and toothpaste. They include all the nonabsorbed sugars ending in -ol: sorbitol, mannitol, xylitol, maltitol. They are also found in apples, apricots, lychee, nashi pears, nectarines, peaches, pears, plums, cauliflower, mushrooms, snow peas, and isomalt.

EAT RIGHT FOR YOUR BLOOD TYPE

Have you heard of this one? Based on a blood type of A, B, AB, or O, there are foods that may or may not sit well with you. Some people have had success following these diets. At first, I wondered how this could be true. Then I looked into it a little. The theory is that the gene that codes your blood type affects nearby genes that code for other factors. In clinic, I've found that most people with O blood type do better on a diet that includes meat, while vegetarians are often the ones with A or B blood types. But that's just my observation. Laura Power, PhD, published in the Townsend Letter for Doctors in June 1991. Dr. Power found important interactions between blood type and dietary lectin. (Lectins are actually used in the lab to diagnose those with type A blood.) When people with a sensitive gastro lining consume lectins to excess, it can cause intestinal damage, disrupt digestion, and lead to nutritional deficiencies (malabsorption). Lectins are prevalent in grains and (especially undercooked) beans such as kidney and lima.

Curious as I am, I read Peter D'Adamo's book *Eat Right for Your Blood Type* (https://www.dadamo.com). Apparently, there is plenty of science to back up the concept of using your blood type to direct your food choices. According to the theory, O blood types do better with paleo-style diets. Type As are better with a macrobiotic, vegetarian, or vegan. They typically do well with soy, while others do not. Type Bs are more Mediterranean or pesco-vegetarian. Bs do well with dairy. Types B and AB have many odd issues with foods such as chicken and corn (hint: it's the lectins). *Eat Right for Your Blood Type* is based on the evolution of our ancestors, where they lived, and what they ate. If you like this idea, get the book and learn more. You can try to eat according to your blood type. A food sensitivity test will help guide your choices and heal your gut.

FASTING

You name it, there is a diet for it. I've mentioned only a few. Most foods are off-limits in some diet or another.

This goes to show there is no one right diet for everyone. Then I asked myself, is there a diet with no food? Apparently yes, there is. It is called fasting (covered more in chapter 8). No shopping, cooking, or meal prep required. You just don't eat anything. First part sounds enticing. That saves a ton of time. But wait. Don't we kind of need food? Ah. Back to the purpose of why we eat. It's for nutrition and energy and building blocks of life-living and life-giving requirements. Oh, yes, it is not just to please the two inches at the top of our digestive track. I am talking about the tongue. What a demanding little creature that taste device can be.

"All kinds of animals, birds, reptiles, and sea creatures are being tamed and have been tamed by mankind, but no human being can tame the tongue. It is a restless evil, full of deadly poison."

—JAMES 3:7

I always thought James was talking about taming the tongue with regard to what we say. Perhaps he was talking about eating, too. Hmm. Well, they do say every time you read any Bible passage, you get something different from it. That's why they call it the living word. Jesus also said we cannot live on bread alone. I don't think he meant gluten. Likely more to do with fasting, right? Feast on the Holy Spirit of divine nature while giving yourself digestive rest. At least that's how I could fast. If I tell myself I am not eating for seventeen or more hours, my inner critic freaks out and I want to eat everything in sight. Oh yeah, that's another diet. Everything I see I eat—the "see food" diet! Sorry, that's an old one but couldn't help it. I digress.

WHEN "CHEATING" MAKES YOU MISERABLE

"Can't you just cheat a little?" my dear friend asks sitting across from me at a restaurant. I used to eat the deep-fried perch as a treat once in a while. To boot, on the way home from the restaurant, there's an old-fashioned dairy. The ice cream there feels like velvet on your tongue. All the flavours. My order? Usually chocolate.

These days, these "treats" are no longer fun. It's not about cheating. I'm not on a diet. It's a choice to feel better. It's about not wanting to be laden with headaches, acne, joint pain, brain fog, burning in my body, congestion, constipation, or diarrhea and fatigue. The treat is to not wake up the next morning feeling like the worst cold or flu ever is about to set in. To not have a bellyache for a month. To go to the bathroom without literally shitting a brick. (Sorry, but it's true!) Even little tastes set me off. The few moments on the lips aren't worth it. Ice-cream amnesia initially set in, and I would let that smooth, cold, creamy taste slide down. Time and time again, I'd be in pain. Not a lactose (gas, bloat, and immediate diarrhea) type of reaction. Pain for days and maybe weeks. Then the feeling, like a cloud of doom, builds up over my head and is going to rain on me at any moment. I believe that's the dairy. Then there's the chocolate. Oh, I love chocolate. I love coffee, too. The taste, the aroma. At least I once did. Younger me would easily drink eight cups in a night to stay up studying so I could pack all I wanted to do into a day. Until migraines like lightning shot through my head. I once spent a week in the hospital. Caffeine—not my birth control, as the doctors suspected—was the cause of my vascular spasms. (Although years later, we learned the pill has its own long-term effects on the gut.) With caffeine, I peak, I crash, then my body is mash. That means tea, coffee, and chocolate. I got away with dark chocolate without the dairy for a while, but even then, eventually it became too stimulating and undid me. Alas, no caffeine for me. Well, maybe a little green tea. It burns slower and has L-Theanine to balance it out. Still, I could be in denial. I know in times of intense stress, I have to put the green tea aside, too. Evidently, it is not cheating to have this stuff. It is not even a treat anymore. Resisting temptation is not easy, and it can take years of trial, error, and most of all, overcoming denial. I say this again: if we are quiet enough in our body, we know what's going on. Listen. What is your body saying to you? Maybe it is telling you something, and you are not listening. Or maybe the messages it sends are a bit confusing.

Below are some guidelines for what to eat. Consider these in light of your food sensitivities (more on testing in the next chapter). When I sit down with someone, we have the daily diet tips (listed below) printed out, then just put a line through the things they are going to avoid for a while or forever. These tips are guidelines for shopping and building your meals. Lots of room to mix and match.

DAILY DIET TIPS

Think of what you eat as building blocks. Legos, for example. Different colours, shapes, and sizes that fit together and create a structure. Here we have six basic blocks: vegetables, fruits, fats, proteins, fibre, carbohydrates. Now, this is a little different than what you might expect. Yes, I do know that fibre and fruit can go hand in hand and that they are indeed both carbohydrates. Also, foods like nuts will fit into three basic categories: fats, carbs, and proteins. Fruits and vegetables are often grouped together in food groups, but I separate them because often people eat too many fruits and barely enough vegetables.

VEGETABLES—SIX TO TEN SERVINGS

If you learn only one thing from this book, let it be to eat more vegetables. All kinds of bright, colourful, fresh, and vibrant vegetables. Organic, if at all possible. Do this, and you too will feel fresh and vibrant. Vegetables offer over 5,000 reasons to eat them, including polyphenols, vitamins, minerals, antioxidants, fibre, flavonoids, phytosterols, and many more plant compounds that provide energy, help us heal, eliminate toxins, and discard our waste.

Start with the brassica family of vegetables. Cruciferous is another name they go by—basically the cabbage family. This wonderful family of vegetables includes kale, collards, arugula, broccoli, cauliflower, brussels sprouts, swiss chard, collard greens, turnips, radishes, radish greens, and kohlrabi. The ultimate goal for the average adult is three cups a day. Lightly steamed or raw, and some roasted or baked. It may seem like a lot if you aren't used to eating these kinds of vegetables. Start low and build up slow. Cruciferous vegetables help the liver detoxify. Throw some raw olive oil and sea salt on them. Yum!

Bitter greens are another category to think about. Bitter food helps stimulate digestion. The Italians typically eat their salad greens after they eat their main meal. Americans tend to have their salad as a first course or with their main meal. Either way, the bitterness helps get the gastric juices flowing. You can acquire a taste for bitter greens. Start with a few nibbles and go from there. You could aim upwards to three cups of leafy greens a day. Less in winter. Too much cold raw food in cold raw weather or in times when digestion is challenged is just too much work for the body. Leafy greens include spinach, romaine, chicory, mustard greens, dandelion, leaf lettuce (red and green), radicchio, endive, and watercress.

Other vegetables to think about for flavour and fibre are celery,

celery root, garlic, onions, zucchini, cucumber, asparagus, fennel, and parsnip. About one cup of these a day is a good bet.

Another group of vegetables is the orange, red, and purple ones: carrots, beets, sweet potato, squash, and peppers. These are generally higher in sugars and therefore sweet. That's why one cup of them counts as a carbohydrate. The orange in vegetables is a sign of beta-carotene. This nutrient converts to vitamin A in the body, which is important for your eyes, skin, and gut lining. It needs an enzyme to convert, and if you genetically miss the boat on this enzyme, too many orange vegetables will literally turn you orange. I know this because it has happened to me! My palms and soles of my feet turn orange when I eat too many carrots. Been there, done that! This is why I take a cod liver oil supplement to naturally get a direct source of vitamin A since my body doesn't convert beta-carotene so well.

All vegetables contain carbohydrates, but the green leafies and the cruciferous ones I don't worry too much about counting as carbs (if you are counting). I find sometimes it is good to understand what a serving is and know how many servings in a day are appropriate to meet your goals. Then, once a routine is established, you will naturally know how to balance your daily intake. The concept of building blocks is great. Blocks of colours are easier to imagine than cups of random vegetables. For example, instead of thinking of a cup of raw broccoli or spinach, imagine one green building block. Start with how many blocks of each you need to have in your day and just ask yourself, "So far today, did I get three light green, three dark green, one orange or red, and some mix of other vegetables?" If not, add a block into your day to make it more complete. When you cook down something like collard greens or spinach, you can pack a whole lot into your day. Just don't eat the same things every day. Not only is this really boring, but it keeps you from getting the variety nature intends you to get. If you barely eat a cup of vegetables a day, start low and slowly build up. Evolution, not revolution. If your digestion is very fragile or elderly, cook most of your vegetables and aim for three cups a day.

A WORD ON OXALATES

I once had a super fit young lady in to see me, and she was aghast to discover she had kidney stones. How could this happen, you ask? She eats well, lives clean, and exercises regularly. Well, if you eat spinach in your smoothie every day for three years, this can totally happen. Spinach is high in oxalates, which are consistent with the formation of one type of kidney stone.

The oxalates also have great binding power not only to form stones but to bind to the other minerals in your diet such as iron. The crystals are sharp and pointy and have the potential to cause pain and inflammation all over the body. Vulvodynia, fibromyalgia, and joint pain are just a few examples of oxalate damage beyond kidney stones.

Takeaway is, spinach is okay, but get some variety. If one week you pick up a bin of spinach to enjoy, next week get arugula instead. Here's a low-oxalate diet to consider for kidney stones: https://kidneystones.uchicago.edu/how-to-eat-a-low-oxalate-diet/.

Beyond diet, the microbiome does play a role in the absorption and secretion of oxalates. The presence of a naturally occurring oxalate degrading bacteria, *Oxalobacter formigenes* (*Oxf*), and certain strains of *Lactobacillus* and *Bifidobacterium* help reduce oxalate absorption.[71] It is more than just this handful of bacteria that do the job. A balanced microbiome with broad diversity of healthy species tends to help the most.[72]

To summarize, nature has packed a powerful punch in the plant kingdom. Many plants offer one or more of these 5,000 nutritional perks:

- Defend against bacteria, virus, mold, fungi, and parasites
- Protect against chronic disease, including cardiovascular disease, neurodegeneration, and cancer
- Purify and renew the blood
- Nourish
- Cleanse the body of toxins
- Some have stimulating effects, others relaxing effects
- Anti-inflammatory
- Provide natural soil microbes
- Heal the gut

FATS—FOUR TO SIX SERVINGS

I will keep this pretty simple. Your brain is nearly 60 percent fat. Each and every cell in your body has a membrane that is made of a lot of fats. Cell membrane or "mem-brain"? Think of it like a brain choosing what goes in and out. Eat the good fats, and the

71 Mehta, M., Goldfarb, D. S., & Nazzal, L. (2016). The role of the microbiome in kidney stone formation. *International Journal of Surgery*, 36(Pt D), 607–612. https://doi.org/10.1016/j.ijsu.2016.11.024

72 Lee, J. A., & Stern, J. M. (2019). Understanding the link between gut microbiome and urinary stone disease. *Current Urology Reports*, 20(5), 19. https://doi.org/10.1007/s11934-019-0882-8

membrane is fluid and allows nutrients to flow in and waste to flow out. Eat too many bad fats, and the membrane gets rigid. A rigid membrane makes it difficult to get nutrients in and waste out. Rule of thumb: If your carbs are low, keep fats high, and vice versa.

There is a class of fats called essential fatty acids (EFAs); omega-3 and omega-6 are essential to us because our bodies cannot make them out of other things we eat. We have to take them in directly. Omega-3s are found in cold-water fatty fish such as mackerel, herring, salmon, and sardines. Animal-based omega-3s are much easier for the body to use than plant-based omega-3s from hemp, walnuts, chia, and flax. In most, omega-3s convert to DHA (docosahexaenoic acid) and EPA (eicosapentaenoic acid). Premature infants and some adults with diabetes or high blood pressure may struggle to make the EPA and DHA.[73] Direct supplementation may be necessary for those with diseases or poor diets.

Both omega-3 and omega-6 provide benefits. Typically, we look in the diet for a ratio of five or six omega-6s to one omega-3. The North American diet often has a ratio more like 20:1. A bit out of whack, wouldn't you say? Especially if you consider that during evolution, the paleolithic days, the ratio was more like 1:1. So try to get more of omega-3s and less omega-6s. Why? High omega-6 intake is linked to obesity, atherosclerosis, and diabetes. Omega-6s are found in industrial seed oils (canola, corn, soy, safflower). In fact, they are found in almost all plants *except* coconut, palm, and cocoa. Omega-6 has something called linoleic acid (LA). The body turns this into arachidonic acid (AA), an inflam-

73 Simopoulos, A. P. (2016). An increase in the omega-6/omega-3 fatty acid ratio increases the risk for obesity. *Nutrients, 8*(3), 128. https://doi.org/10.3390/nu8030128

mation and blood clot promoter. You also get AA direct from peanuts, grain-fed meats, dairy, and eggs. Balance your fat intake.

Omega-9s are good, too. That's basically olive, cashew, avocado, and almond oils. It drives me nuts when people buy capsules or supplements of omega-9. For goodness sake, just put a tablespoon or two on your vegetables. This will help you absorb their fat-soluble nutrients, vitamins A, D, E, and K.

In addition to omega-3-6-9 fats, there are MCT or medium-chain triglycerides. These are found in coconut oil. Initially, they were thought to negatively affect cholesterol levels in the body. Subsequent research revealed this not to be the case. It is really easy for the body to use MCTs for energy. It is the pride of the keto diet and can be very useful for diabetics who are insulin sensitive.

A daily intake of healthy fats might look like:

- two tablespoons raw olive oil
- two tablespoons of coconut oil
- one-quarter to one-half avocado
- one-quarter to one-half cup of nuts and seeds (nuts are also a carbohydrate source laden with fibre)
- one to three teaspoons of fish oil. This can come from a serving of freshwater fish (sardines, salmon, mackerel, or herring) or from a supplement. If taking a supplement, always look for one that is third-party tested and cleansed of heavy metals. I think the cod liver oil liquid is the most natural you can get. The more they modify the fat molecule, the less natural it is.

What about the fat with meats? It's likely best to trim the fat on your meat, especially if heart disease and high cholesterol run in your family.

Cheese? Generally, you're looking at a lot of saturated fat. It's not as high in protein as you might think. Cottage cheese is the best protein bet.

Please eat some of the skin on your chicken. It provides necessary choline, a building block for acetylcholine, an important part of a healthy nervous system function.

If you have had your gallbladder removed or have issues with the function of the gallbladder or have a traffic jam (blockage) in the duct, then you will need to eat fats in small bits throughout the day. Bile is like dish soap. It breaks the fat down into little drops. You can see this if you put a greasy pan into the dishwater. The suds disappear, and there are a million little globules floating on the surface. A clear indicator of poor digestion of fats is something else that floats: your stool. If you have complete blockage in the gallbladder ducts, your stool will be white and floating. Warning: this happens early and often with those sensitive to gluten.

Enough about fats. What about protein?

PROTEIN

How much do you really need, and where does it come from? Protein is found in meat, nuts and seeds, lentils and beans, fish, chicken, eggs, and dairy. You can estimate your protein requirements at 0.8 g/kg of body weight for the average person. Runners and body builders might need more like 1 g/kg. This works out to average of 50–100 g per day for most women and 60–130 g per day for most men. Some days, you might get more protein than others. This is okay. We are not meant to feast every day. You might ask about animal versus plant protein. Yes and yes. Both are important. We are designed to be omnivores—plant- and meat eaters. People with blood type O tend to do better with more meat in their diet, whereas those with AB tend to do better with more plant-based diets. Animal-based protein offers complete protein in one meal, whereas plant-based will combine over the day to balance things out. But you have to eat a variety. When your gut is compromised, you may find it easier to break down plant-based protein, which means for a short time you eat less animal-based foods, or when you do eat them, cook them really slow and long (slow roast or slow cooked) so your body gets some help breaking the protein down.

List of High-Protein Foods and Amount of Protein in Each
Animal Proteins

Beef	Hamburger patty, 4 oz: 28 g Steak, 6 oz: 42 g Most cuts of beef: 7 g of protein per ounce
Chicken	Chicken breast, 3.5 oz: 30 g Chicken thigh: 10 g (for average size)
Pork	Pork chop, average: 22 g Pork loin or tenderloin, 4 oz: 29 g
Fish	Most fish fillets or steaks, about 22 g of protein for 3 oz: 22 g Tuna, 6 oz can: 40 g

Plant Proteins

Beans	Most beans (black, pinto, lentils, etc.) about 7-10 g protein per half cup of cooked beans Split peas, 1 cup cooked: 8 g *Soy milk, 1 cup: 6-10 g *Soybeans, 1 cup cooked: 14 g *Note: Most Caucasian people do not have the enzymes to properly digest soy.
Nuts and Seeds ½ cup servings	Almonds: 8 g Cashews: 5 g Pecans: 2.5 g Sunflower seeds: 6 g Pumpkin seeds: 8 g Flax seeds: 8 g Hemp hearts: 12 g

Avoid peanuts as they promote arachidonic acid cycle, which leads to inflammation. Peanuts also are prone to molds, which, when it comes to candida overgrowth, can be a challenge. Fungi and molds are like cousins, and they like to hang out together. If you battle candida overgrowth, aka big sugar cravings, avoid the peanut butter for a while. You might be able to add it back in and have in small amounts later. Note that a lot of peanut butters on the market have sugar and added industrial seed fats, compounding the inflammatory factors. When you do go for peanut butter, get the natural kind with nothing added.

Eggs and Dairy

Egg, Large	1 egg: 6 g (2 eggs is one serving of protein)
Milk	1 cup: 8 g
Cottage Cheese	½ cup: 15 g
Yogurt	1 cup: Usually 8-12 g

Many people with gut issues have problems digesting dairy. Dairy is made up of sugars, proteins, and fats. Some people can't tolerate lactose. That's the sugar. Lactose intolerance is classically the pain, gas, bloat, and almost-immediate diarrhea that comes after eating dairy products. Lactose-intolerant people can usually get away with a little milk or cream in their tea or coffee, some hard cheeses, and full-fat yogurt. Lots of times, something is labelled "dairy-free" when it is actually just lactose-free. There is a difference because some people are protein intolerant, which means whey and casein are likely the things causing problems; lactose-free products are of no help and the pain in the stomach is less bloat and more ache. If you are lactose-, casein-, and whey sensitive, then you get the whole enchilada of symptoms. Note that gluten-sensitive people often grow an intolerance to milk protein as well because of the cross-reaction of proteins. Not too many are sensitive to the milk fat, which is why lots of people can consume ghee, or clarified butter. Ghee is butter without any of the milk proteins or sugars. Eating dairy-free margarine is about as good as eating plastic and food dye. Trust me, it won't provide any nutritional benefit—and the jury is out on whether it will do any harm. It certainly will if you are sensitive to yellow food dye, which many are. Really, our body is not meant to break down those manufactured chemicals.

FERMENTED FOODS

Fermented foods offer added benefits to the microbiome and are consumed around the world. Over the centuries, various cultures—Asian, European, and North American—found ways of eating food that had "gone bad." Once they found out the fermented food was okay to eat, they used bacterial cultures to ferment food on purpose to help preserve it.

Fermented milk becomes yogurt or kefir. Kefir is more liquid than yogurt and holds three times as many bacteria. The travellers through the Caucasus Mountains between Europe and Asia figured that out. Kimchi is fermented vegetables, a traditional Korean fermented food that typically includes cabbage and other vegetables, garlic, ginger, hot pepper, salt, and sometimes fish sauce. Chinese and Japanese found soybeans (often mixed with wheat, barley, or rice) ferment to make natto, miso, tempeh, or soy sauce (because of the wheat or barley, these are to be avoided on a gluten-free diet). Sauerkraut is fermented cabbage of German heritage. Cheese is fermented in many different cultures. And speaking of culture, a group of bacteria used in fermentation is called a culture, except in kombucha (fermented tea and juice); its culture is called SCOBY because it is a symbiotic culture of bacteria and yeast. Other well-known fermented beverages include beer and wine. In small quantities, these can be medicinal, too. You learned earlier that red wine in small quantities can improve the health of the microbiome. However, too much alcohol of any kind will deplete the microbiome. The key takeaway? Add a little culture to your life with some of these fermented foods. However, don't do so if you are in the process of resetting the gut, as you will have to be careful of the unknown microbes you may introduce. The guidance on that will be individual and perhaps even on a trial-and-error basis.

A good friend tells me of a woman at church who makes sourdough bread from a culture that is over 70 years old. Apparently, even people who cannot eat gluten can eat her bread. Some celiac people have tried it and tolerate it okay. I say this culture needs to be grown, protected (likely patented), and studied! Who knows, just because humans don't have the proper enzymes to digest gluten, maybe it was the yeast all along that digested it for us. Perhaps now, our modern yeast cultures are too bland and no longer break down the wheat proteins. This may explain why we could once tolerate wheat so much better than we can today. Now, wouldn't that be something!

IRON

Heme iron is the most easily absorbed kind and comes only from animals, though animal sources contain both heme and non-heme iron. Iron from animals is seven times more absorbable than plant-based iron. The best source of iron is liver. It is also in other red meat, oysters, and chicken. If you need more iron in your diet and you have troubles taking an iron supplement (they're known to cause constipation) and you don't like or can't get liver, try a pure source of desiccated liver in a capsule.

Heme and iron are important for red blood cell building and provide oxygen to every cell in the body, including those in the gut. Your body will absorb what iron it needs from food if the gastro lining is healthy. If you'd like to increase your iron, it helps to cook in cast iron cookware or throw a "lucky iron fish" in your soup pot. A lucky iron fish is a cast iron kitchen gadget in the shape of a fish. You don't eat it; you just put it into your pot so the liquid can absorb iron.

Non-heme sources such as red teff grain, blackstrap molasses, white beans, and dark chocolate are still valid, though less absorbable. Foods with vitamin C, like bell peppers or citrus fruits, help you absorb heme iron better. Oxalates, phytates, phosphates, and tannates prevent iron absorption. This is why the iron in spinach doesn't get absorbed so well. It is blocked by the high levels of oxalates.

CARBOHYDRATES

Carbohydrates start to get digested in the mouth with chewing and salivary enzymes. Usually, they do it by removing a chemical group or bending it around to change its structure, which is very helpful in speeding up digestion. A carbohydrate provides the body mostly with energy and also with some structure.

Carbohydrates are found in nuts, seeds, vegetables, grains, rice, fruits, syrups, sweeteners, honey, and alcohol. They are abundant in processed and packaged goods. That includes just about anything found in the middle aisle of the grocery store: cereal, bread, jams, sauces, beans, lentils, soups, chips, soda pop, ice cream, breading on frozen foods, pizza, pasta, tortillas. The list goes on. It is often helpful to focus on what *to* eat instead of what *not* to eat. We'll do just that. Not all carbohydrates are bad. Most people do fine with modest amounts.

Insulin sensitivity and *Candida* overgrowth in the gut are two very good reasons for carbohydrate restriction. Keto diets are helpful here. When we do the gut reboot, early stages are very much like a keto diet or whole foods or sugar detox diet. If you are sensitive to FODMAPs, you may have difficulty with certain carbohydrates. Elaine Gottschall's book *Breaking the Vicious Cycle* explains how the gut breaks down different types of carbs. If you are interested in that level of detail, I highly recommend reading it.

FIBRE

Fibre is part of carbohydrates. Whole grain wheat products are a great source of fibre. However, many people have gluten-related disorders (known or unknown), and that's why I advocate gluten-free sources of fibre. That said, someone on a gluten-free diet needs to take extra care to get enough fibre. Fibre is a part of plant cells and is not absorbed by the body. Remember, North Americans typically get 2–4 g per day; the goal is around 30 g. Build yours up slowly!

Most plant sources deliver both soluble and insoluble fibres. These delay entry of carbohydrates/sugars into the bloodstream, improving blood glucose management. When selecting your carbohydrates, be sure to include some soluble and insoluble sources of fibre.

Soluble

Soluble fibre forms a gel that helps heal the gut lining and delays stomach emptying, helping you feel full sooner. Soluble fibre traps and excretes cholesterol, preventing it from recirculating. Soluble fibres to eat daily include Medjool dates, pectin, lentils, apples, oranges, pears, gluten-free oats, strawberries, nuts, flaxseeds, beans, dried peas, blueberries, psyllium, cucumbers, celery, and carrots.

Insoluble

Insoluble fibre bulks the stool and clears out toxins. Include some best sources daily: vegetables and fruit in general, especially acorn squash, peas, brussels sprouts, unsweetened coconut, kale and zucchini, raspberries, blackberries, and pears.

How many carbohydrates do you really need? It depends on your state of health and activity level. Less than 50 g per day is very low carb. You will get this from some vegetables and nuts and seeds alone. Or 1 fruit, ½ cup nuts, and ½ cup oats. To stick to this long term is extremely difficult and not necessarily healthy. A daily intake of 50–75 g for women or 65–100 g for men takes some dedication, but it can be done.

Most would do well with a moderate carbohydrate intake. However, in the early stages of gut reset, it will be necessary to be very low carbohydrate for a short time, then migrate to low carb and eventually maintain a moderate intake.

Each serving of carbohydrates is 15 g. You could find that in a tablespoon of maple syrup, so watch it! Packaged and processed foods are notorious for hidden sugars. Look at the labels! How much is a serving? How many carbs in that? Once you start reading labels, you will see how much better it is to get your carbs from whole foods. Plus, there are all sorts of sugars, additives, salt, food dyes, and chemicals in processed food. Think about it. These are foods that have to last on the shelf for a while without going bad.

Sugar and noncaloric artificial sweeteners (stevia, saccharin, sucralose, and aspartame) change the composition of the gut microbiome and can lead to cardiovascular disease and glucose intolerance.[74] If you want to play with the diabetes fire, here's one way it starts.

74   Suez, J., Korem, T., Zeevi, D., Zilberman-Schapira, G., Thaiss, C. A., Maza, O., Israeli, D., Zmora, N., Gilad, S., Weinberger, A., Kuperman, Y., Harmelin, A., Kolodkin-Gal, I., Shapiro, H., Halpern, Z., Segal, E., & Elinav, E. (2014). Artificial sweeteners induce glucose intolerance by altering the gut microbiota. *Nature*, 514(7521), 181–186. https://doi.org/10.1038/nature13793

I said we would focus on what *to* eat, and I am going to keep that promise. Focus on the following five groups of carbohydrates: fruits, nuts and seeds, lentils dried (cooked) beans, starchy root vegetables, and gluten-free grains. If you had two servings a day from each of the five groups, that's a moderate carbohydrate intake at 75 g for the day. Yes, variety is important.

Serving sizes listed below:

Fruit: one to two servings per day

- one small apple, orange, banana, pear, peach, or kiwi
- ¾ cup pineapple
- ½ small mango, papaya, or grapefruit
- one cup of berries
- 1¼ c of melon
- 12 cherries, 17 grapes, 4 apricots, 2 small plums
- one large tomato

Lentils, dried (cooked) beans and peas

- ⅓ cup hummus
- ½ cup cooked black, garbanzo, kidney, navy, lima, pinto, white beans, lentils, black-eyed or split peas

Nuts and seeds

- ½ cup = 1 serving

Starchy and root vegetables

- one small or ½ large baked potato
- one cup butternut or acorn squash or pumpkin
- ½ cup sweet potato, yam or cassava, or turnip
- ¼ cup carrots or beets or parsnips

*Certified gluten-free wheat alternatives

- ½ cup cooked oats or buckwheat
- ½ cup quinoa or quinoa flour
- ⅓ cup white or brown rice
- 10 Mary's (Gone) Crackers
- ⅓ cup teff or sorghum flour
- ½ cup coconut flour
- ⅛ cup arrowroot or tapioca flour

*Be sure to buy certified gluten-free to avoid cross-contamination. Even then, some people may find grains in general do not sit well with them. This is where layering on your food sensitivities will really help.

Stay away from the sauces and dips. Ketchup is basically sugar. Plain mustard might work for some, but be really careful if you are gluten sensitive. I'll never forget a trip to our friend's place for the weekend. She is a condiment queen. There were ten different mustards in her fridge. After reading all the labels, I found one that didn't have mustard flour, which is usually contaminated with gluten. Look for the ground mustard seed—that's best. Other than that, use olive oil or coconut oil and some sea salt—maybe some herbs and spices to make your food taste good. A few slices of roasted apples or pears with cinnamon as a condiment may also be nice. Or some fermented vegetables. Enough with the sugar-laden goop!

At this point, you may feel unsupported in the food choice changes. Sure, it is great to have building blocks, but how do you turn the food into recipes that make a great tasting meal? Use garlic, onion, parsley, sage, rosemary, thyme, basil, oregano, chili, paprika, celery seed, salt, pepper, ginger, cardamom, cinnamon, turmeric, curry, and mint as your kitchen helpers. There are plenty of paleo, allergen-free, grain-free, keto, or Mediterranean-style cookbooks out there.

Now, you might wonder why you need to go gluten-free. I highly recommend it. None of us has the enzymes to properly break down gluten. If you have digestive challenges, chances are you have lost your oral tolerance to it. When proper testing is done, 70 percent of people have sensitivity (elevated antibodies) to wheat. Once the inflammatory cascade sets up, your chance for autoimmunity increases. The biggest organ affected by wheat is not the gut but the brain.

Finally, a really good reason to stay away from gluten while healing the gut is that whole grains are super hard on the digestive tract. They can shred anyone's gut. Most people's will heal in twenty minutes or so. But for those with a compromised gut lining, inflammation in the gastrointestinal tract and/or a sensitivity to gluten, it can take up to five hours to heal. Then it's lunchtime.

I have to say, after being away from gluten so long and now that there are so many alternatives, I don't really miss it. You adapt.

You get creative with recipes. Once you start feeling better, why go back to feeling terrible again?

Ugh, but then comes having to call the host of a party. Even after years of dealing with dietary restrictions, I find this difficult. Innately, I am a people pleaser, and it is not like me to expect others to please me. I still have some ounces of guilt calling the host of an intimate dinner party to tell them I have a gluten intolerance and cannot tolerate any dairy. If I gave them the whole list—no gluten, no dairy, no sugar, no soy, no chocolate, no oats, no buckwheat, no teff, no nutritional yeast...You can't imagine the variety of food that people try to make to satisfy these conditions. I stick to a very simple guideline of whole food, no sauces, just olive oil, salt, and pepper, and that works. Or I offer to bring my own. See the appendix for an effective way to contact a hall in advance of an event. Holiday season is a bit of a nightmare. Dinner parties and cocktail events are like land mines. I usually end up losing weight because most places we go, I can't eat anything. As an alternative, we've tried not to go places. That's one solution but a very boring lonely existence. Now I try to eat a little before going and just do my best at the event. That can work if I focus on the people and not the food. So long as the people don't focus on the food, I am not eating!

Sometimes I feel like I've become "that" person. That needy, "look at me" kind of gal. Ugh. I am not doing this because it is glorious. It's not a fad or passing fancy. I cannot eat gluten (or other things) because it makes me SICK. Not just for a day or so but for many days. Additionally, research shows that even having gluten exposure once a month increases a celiac or non-celiac gluten-sensitive person's risk of death. If for a moment those kind, well-intentioned hosts could feel what I feel when I've eaten gluten or dairy, they would be so thankful they don't have to concern themselves with this every meal. Then there are the other guests. Generally, they won't be too happy about getting a "gluten- and dairy-free" meal. Gluten, dairy, and sugar are in so many tasty recipes, let's face it. Over time, I have grown to love my diet. It keeps the inflammation down, keeps me from feeling sick, and keeps my brainpower at its optimum. So yes, plain food is great, thank you. See how grumpy I get with this? Am I angry? Maybe a little. There is always more to work on.

You still may not be sure where to start. Use the Diet Diary tool (see appendix) to track your diet and how you feel for a week. Then start to focus on one of the building blocks. Or focus on one meal at a time. Exchange your existing habits and meal options. Essentially, change one bite at a time. Make a new diet diary with coloured pens. For example, use green, red, and orange for the correspondingly coloured vegetables, yellow for fats, pink for protein, and brown for carbs. Even if you focus on one colour at a time, that's great. It's about progress, not perfection.

When you are ready, turn the page, and we'll take a deeper look at the foods you might be sensitive to and what's actually going on in your gut!

A DEEPER LOOK

Here's what you'll learn in this chapter:

- Microbiome analysis—how healthy is *your* gut?
- Types of food sensitivity testing
- Other tests that can be helpful for gut health
- Patient examples so you get a sense of why these tests are important

Ever stop to look in the mirror? Not in a vain way, but so you can adjust your jacket collar, check if you have spinach in your teeth, or fix your hair after you pulled a sweater over your head?

For the same reasons we might need to look in the mirror from time to time, we may choose to run some tests. It gives you a chance to get a glimpse of yourself in a way you can't by just looking down and around. Sometimes we can get a better picture of what's going on by standing back and taking a full-length view. This makes it a lot easier to decide what needs adjusting.

As the businessman Jack Welch said, "You can't change what you can't measure."

Laboratory tests can help confirm what your body tries to tell you. Symptoms can result from many different problems. Take a headache, for example. Did you hit your head, get a hangover, drink too much coffee, or try to quit smoking cold turkey? Is the weather changing? Are your sinuses stuffed full? Is your hat too tight? Or do you have leaky gut? Is gram-negative bacterial overgrowth off-gassing toxins that result in an inflammatory cascade that causes your headache?

Another example: you have a stomachache after eating a pizza. Was it the cheese, the crust, the tomatoes, or the pepperoni that caused it? Maybe cheese and the crust? How would you know? Eat bread alone. Eat cheese alone. Wait and see. But maybe it was the soda pop you drank with it? Or do you have lead contamination? Sometimes we just don't know. And how else will we determine the balance of the bugs in our gut? We can't just vomit the contents and get the calculator out. It doesn't work that way.

It does work to do some special tests available through your naturopathic or functional medicine doctor. The top three specialty tests for gut health are:

1. Comprehensive stool analysis with parasitology
2. Wheat and gluten sensitivity testing
3. Reliable food sensitivity test

Sure, there are a lot of other very helpful tests, but I think if we know your symptoms and know what's going on with these three, then we can make a pretty good plan to move forward. Now, tests cost money and are not always covered by health insurance or benefit plans. You might balk at how expensive they are, but I want you to think about this for a minute. What have you spent your money on in the past week? An $8 coffee? Twenty-four dollars at the fast-food window? One hundred twenty dollars on supplements you thought might be helpful? Five hundred dollars for a gym membership you haven't used in (admit it) a very long time? Amazon adventures? Prioritize your health. It's the best thing you can do.

Laboratory tests evolve and improve over time with technological and scientific advances. Ask your practitioner if they have the most up-to-date version of a given test.

COMPREHENSIVE STOOL ANALYSIS AND PARASITOLOGY

Examples of comprehensive stool tests currently on the market:

1. GI 360: https://www.gi360.com
2. GIMAP: https://www.diagnosticsolutionslab.com/tests/gi-map

Remember, a healthy regular stool is not always indicative of a healthy microbiome. Stool analysis tells you what bacteria, parasites, and fungi make up your microbiome; how well you digest your food; whether you show markers of inflammation; and how healthy your colon is. It reveals how well the microflora in your gut are working for you by measuring microbiome by-products for fermentation, otherwise known as short-chain fatty acids (SCFAs).

SCFAs are by-products of fermenting food fibre in the gut. These acids fend off infection and disease. SCFAs also increase the availability of calcium and magnesium[75] and feed the cells lining the gut. Depletion of SCFAs is found in people with inflammatory bowel disease. Microbes need fibre to ferment to make SCFAs, and this test shows whether your gut provides enough fibre and the right balance of microbes.

INFLAMMATORY MARKERS

A rise in inflammatory markers may indicate infection or inflammatory bowel disease. These markers include calprotectin, lactoferrin, lysozyme, secretory IgA, white blood cells, and mucus.

BETA-GLUCURONIDASE

Some bacteria (*Lactobacillus* and *Enterococcus*) make beta-glucuronidase. This substance can remove the "packing tape" the liver uses when it prepares toxins for removal from the body. A result of higher levels of beta-glucuronidase, toxic environmental forms of estrogens (e.g., from plastic, pesticides, or insecticides) can recirculate back into the body. It is projected that the more recirculation of estrogens meant for export, the greater the risk of estrogen-positive cancers such as breast, ovary, and uterine. Higher levels of Beta-glucuronidase in older adults are also related to colon cancer[76] and other gastrointestinal cancers.[77]

75 O'Callaghan, A., & van Sinderen, D. (2016). Bifidobacteria and their role as members of the human gut microbiota. *Frontiers in Microbiology, 7*, 925. https://doi.org/10.3389/fmicb.2016.00925

76 Kim, D. H., & Jin, Y. H. (2001). Intestinal bacterial beta-glucuronidase activity of patients with colon cancer. *Archives of Pharmacal Research, 24*(6), 564-567. https://doi.org/10.1007/BF02975166

77 Khanolkar, M. M., Sirsat, A. V., Walvekar, S. S., Bhansali, M. S., & Desouza, L. J. (1997). Modified method for determination of serum beta-glucuronidase: A comparative study using P-nitrophenyl glucuronide and phenolphthalein glucuronide as substrate in gastrointestinal tract carcinomas. *Indian Journal of Clinical Biochemistry, 12*(1), 67-70. https://doi.org/10.1007/BF02867959

WHEAT AND GLUTEN SENSITIVITY TESTING

Sam is 70 years old, a retired physiotherapist, and father of two daughters. He suffers a stroke and loses the ability to walk, and his memory degenerates. His wife, Sue, does most of the communication for him as Sam is slow to respond and can't complete his sentences. Sam has had lifelong issues with constipation. He never thought much of it, just took laxatives daily to compensate. When he first visits me, he limps in with a cane. Sue comes with him. His intake and family medical history reveals his two daughters are both celiac, and neither he nor his wife had ever been tested. Celiac disease is passed down genetically from the mom or dad to the child. If children or parents test positive, guess who else ought to be tested? Now, Sam doesn't seem to think he had that much of a problem with bread or gluten. Nonetheless, we order in the Cyrex Array 3 kit and went ahead with the test, which involves sending a blood sample to Cyrex Laboratories for analysis. The report comes back in about three weeks. It is important to consider your symptoms alongside the test results. A seasoned practitioner can help you make appropriate lifestyle and dietary decisions.

Back to Sam. He is just fine for the markers conventional medicine would examine. The tissue transglutaminase and antigliadin antibody markers are totally normal. But the markers that indicate gluten ataxia are not normal. Ataxia means a lack of muscle control due to damaged neurons in the base of the brain. Sam is surprised but willing to try a gluten-free diet to see how he'd do. Sue was accustomed to preparing gluten-free meals for their girls, so she is on board.

Six weeks later, Sam walks into my office. He has no cane. The difference is incredible. His mind is sharper, too. He can speak for himself and carry on a conversation. "Keep up the gluten-free, and I'll see you in another six weeks," I tell him. The next time we catch up, he is low in mood and visibly upset. He doesn't think the gluten-free diet is working anymore. He's been feeling unsteady on his feet lately, and he doesn't like it. Sue jabs him in the ribs and says, "*Come on, Sam, tell Dr. Laura what you've been up to.*" He doesn't budge. She gives him the eye. You know, the "I mean business" look wives give husbands. "*You know. Toronto...*" Sam lets out a big sigh. Then he spills his guts. Turns out, Sam was so excited to be feeling as good as he was that when relatives came to visit, he went and did something he hadn't been able to do for the past four years: a sight-seeing trip culminating in the CN Tower edge walk. That's when a daring person harnesses up and does the world's highest walk on a five-foot ledge about 1,168 ft (116 storeys) above the ground.

"Sam," I say, "*you know we all have our limits. I think you pushed yours a little over the edge. You'll rebound, and you will have to learn your limits and stick 'withinits.'*" Sam reluctantly agrees I might be right. I mean really, I don't just wave a magic wand and boom, you are healed. Your body does the healing, and it can take a little time. Sometimes much longer than we'd wish or hope for.

If Sam had never done the testing, he'd never have found the conviction to go gluten-free. Sometimes people have to see things on a paper with their name on it and colours, charts, and numbers glaring at them before they believe what's going on in their body. They are not quiet in their body. They ignore it whenever possible.

Then there's Penelope. Penelope suffered from fibromyalgia

and irritable bowel syndrome (IBS). She doubted the severity of her gluten intolerance. There is an actomyosin layer in the gut lining—the muscle fibres that give the wave-like motion to move the contents along. When the immune system arms itself against the gluten, the similar protein structure in the gut lining gets mistaken for the gluten, and inflammation and damage results. Now, there are many more places in the body that have similar muscle structure, and the immune system can target them, too. This is why the muscle pains and aches wander around. I wish Penelope's story had a happy ending. Although she tried to be gluten-free for the most part and felt better when she did, she frequently "treated" herself with things such as homemade pasta and birthday cake. She didn't do any gluten or wheat testing to strengthen her conviction. Penelope died from complications of chronic inflammatory conditions, including metabolic and cardiovascular disease. It is sad to lose such a beautiful soul.

Gluten is just one of over a hundred proteins in wheat. Every time any of us eats gluten, some damage is done to the small intestinal lining. For most people, it recovers and repairs in about twenty minutes. For those who are genetically susceptible, it may take up to five hours. Then the next meal comes. Over time, repeated meals containing gluten repeat the damage, with little time for repair and recovery. Eventually, the body cannot keep up. Some trigger point of stress or illness may increase the recovery time. Not everyone has the typical symptoms of fatigue, weight gain, bowel issues, pain, gas, or bloating.

A lot of gastroenterologists know how to screen for celiac disease. They'll typically test for antibodies to alpha-gliadin, transglutaminase-2, and maybe if they're up to date with the scientific literature, they'll also screen for antibodies to deamidated gliadin and endomysium. If some of these tests are positive, then they might do a biopsy to determine if there is damage to the small intestine. If the tests are negative, the patient is generally told that they don't have celiac or gluten intolerance, and that's as far as it goes. Unfortunately, that's not as far as it goes.

Tissue transglutaminase has three different types. Most tests look at only type 2. There is also type 3, which is primarily found in the skin, and type 6, which is primarily found in the brain and nervous system. What's more, type 2 isn't just for the villi in the small intestine. It exists as a layer of protection for all organs—your blood-brain barrier, your liver, your spleen, you name it. That means if your TTG2 is positive and your endoscopic test is negative, you are still reacting to gluten. It's just not in your gut but somewhere else. Most often, it is the brain.

If this is you, the gluten you eat may affect your brain or your skin, or maybe your muscle, but conventional testing will miss this. Take Sam or Penelope, for example. I emphasize, just because the two markers your conventional doc tests for come back negative, *it does not mean you are free from wheat-related damage.*

If you have irritable bowels, diarrhea, bloating, foggy brain, thyroid problems, gallstones, bone, joint, or muscle problems, elevated liver enzymes, osteoporosis, fibromyalgia, depression, anxiety, Parkinson's, ADHD/ADD, or schizophrenia, it is wise to evaluate several critical components of wheat that may contribute to your condition.

Jeanie is another example. Jeanie has multiple sclerosis and is over her healthy weight. When Jeanie first came in to see me, she had a real addiction to sugar. She loves to bake, and that means not only a lot of sugar but gluten, too. Over the past four months, she has made some significant progress. It wasn't overnight. We took it slow, as a process of evolution, not revolution. First, she switched her after-work snack to an apple and twenty almonds. The next month, she observed how much sugar she was actually eating, and each time she had something to eat, she did her best to make a healthier choice. This past month, she tried to remove as much gluten and sugar as she could. In three months, she lost 12 pounds. Now she feels so much more energetic. This is a great example of evolutionary choices. Six months later, Jeanie says, *"I have been following your diet suggestions for my MS (no dairy, no gluten, and have cut back my sugar intake) and have been feeling great. I have lost 26 pounds, and the bloated, 'yucky' feeling (I often lived with but didn't realize how bad it was until it actually went away) is gone."*

One step at a time, and you too will get there. If you are sensitive to gluten and eat a lot of sugar, often the extra weight is inflammatory weight. Stop eating it, and you will get the inflammation down.

Gluten sensitivity plays a role in things such as:

- Attention deficit hyperactivity disorder (ADHD)
- Autism
- Schizophrenia
- Cerebellar ataxia
- Depression
- Anxiety

- Fertility
- Autoimmunity
- Celiac disease
- Gallbladder issues
- Parkinson's disease
- Alzheimer's disease[78]
- Epilepsy and seizures[79]
- Dermatitis herpetiformis
- Polymyalgia
- Osteoporosis
- Liver disease
- Thyroid disease

For more information, visit https://www.cyrexlabs.com or https://www.vibrant-wellness.com/tests/wheat-zoomer/ or talk with your dedicated healthcare provider.

Is it always wheat or gluten? No. Will eliminating gluten alone always fix the issue? No.

How can you know what foods are bothering you? Good question. That's what we are going to talk about next.

FOOD SENSITIVITY TESTING

There are different types of tests available to help you understand what foods your body is reacting to. It can be difficult to tease it

---

78 Daulatzai, M. A. (2015). Non-celiac gluten sensitivity triggers gut dysbiosis, neuroinflammation, gut-brain axis dysfunction, and vulnerability for dementia. *CNS & Neurological Disorders Drug Targets*, 14(1), 110–131. https://doi.org/10.2174/1871527314666150202152436

79 Hadjivassiliou, M., & Zis, P. (2019). Gluten sensitivity and epilepsy: A systematic review. *Journal of Neurology*, 266(7), 1557–1565. https://doi.org/10.1007/s00415-018-9025-2

all apart given that a sensitivity reaction can happen anytime from three minutes to three days after you eat a food. And as we learned, when your toxic bucket is full, it's full. Anything you put in that is even mildly reactive can cause you to overflow with reaction. But since you'll eat a number of other things within those three days, how do you figure out which one you're reacting to? The answer is to test. Testing for food sensitivities is very different from testing for food allergies.

Cross-reactions can happen between environmental and food allergies/sensitivities. For example, people sensitive to latex are prone to becoming sensitive to banana, birch pollen, avocado, kiwi, and melon. Those sensitive to ragweed may find they react to cucumber, watermelon, zucchini, honeydew, and cantaloupe. It may mean that during the season of environmental allergy, you reduce consumption of these potentially cross-reacting foods. Wheat sensitivity can lead to sensitivities to dairy protein, chocolate, coffee, and yeast.

The immune system has different divisions, and each does a different job. They are all responsible for differentiating self from not self. As we learned with gluten, sometimes the system makes mistakes, a crossfire happens, and the innocent bystanders (your tissues) get hurt.

The immune system has IgG, IgA, IgM and IgE, and IgD. Hey, that spells GAMED. It is a bit of a game. You can imagine it like a video game if you wish. The IgA is mostly in the gut lining—our first line of defence where we meet a lot of our outside world and decide what's safe and what isn't. It is what rises when there is inflammation in the gut, such as in people with colitis. We measure this with the stool sample. We can also use a blood test to check if the body is making an immune response for the other players in the immune game. The IgM immune defence comes into play when an infection is first detected.

FOOD ALLERGY TESTING

The "E" in IgE is for emergency or "e"-mmediate. This is the scary, sudden response to certain foods. Your throat closes up, you have shortness of breath, eyes get puffy, tongue swells, and you develop an itchy rash and low blood pressure. Repeated exposure will heighten the response, and eventually you will have to carry an EpiPen to give yourself a quick shot of adrenaline to save your life while you get rushed to the hospital. Testing for IgE allergy response is done through blood work occasionally but most typically through skin prick testing in the immunologist's office.

IGG FOOD SENSITIVITY TESTING

Finally, there is the IgG responsible for general surveillance. This is what gets measured in blood-drawn food sensitivity tests. The body will have a high level of response to foods it is sensitive to for up to twenty-one days after ingestion. If you haven't eaten something in a while because it bothers you, it may or may not show up on your test as a food to avoid. Another thing to point out is, if you overeat a certain food, the IgG test may say you are making a lot of antibodies to it. Your body can build up immunity to foods you eat often. You might be okay with these foods but are overloading the system, and the body is telling you to get more variety in your diet. Lay off these foods for a while, or at least reduce your intake of them, and you'll be fine.

Results are not always easy to interpret. This is why in my practice I use the results from this type of testing simply as a tool for a guided elimination diet. One test that is a bit different is the ALCAT test. This internationally recognized test takes each food protein and tests them one by one to measure how your immune system reacts.

Lastly, there is electrodermal screening (EDS) testing. Dr. Voll designed this skin conductance test years ago, and it is quite interesting. EDS works with the energy wave form of the food that is stored in the computer. A mild electrical current is passed through your body, and the computer records your nervous system's response to each food's energy wave. Think of it this way: everything in the universe is energy, and even foods have a unique wave of energy that identifies every one of them. Of course, there are nuances to a food's energy—for example, not every apple is exactly alike, but the main identifiers allow for a range within the results that can be used to see if the food is aggravating to the body at this time.

I remember my first food sensitivity test. Not good. I was feeling terrible at the time. I remember being in the kitchen preparing vegetables, my joints feeling like knives were slicing through them. Sharp, jabbing pain. I could hardly stand up. My bowels were definitely irritable. I'd eat a white potato, and within minutes my shins would itch and I could scratch them till they bled. Tomatoes? A patch of psoriasis on my left forehead. Walnuts? Itchy throat. Sugar? Acne. Cucumbers? Diarrhea. Sunflower seeds? Gut pain. Cheese? Low mood, headache. I had already figured out I was intolerant to gluten five years prior. *What gives now?* I thought. I was touring clinics in town to see where I might set up my practice. I was in one place, and this lady came roaring out into the hallway to greet me. She said she did food sensitivity testing and would give me a test for free. *Sure*, I thought. *What have I got to lose?*

A ton of foods, including all those mentioned above, came up high on the test. When you have a lot of foods test positive, you can be pretty sure you have leaky gut. How could that be? Gluten contamination? Maybe. How about gut imbalance? *Candida albicans* overgrowth? Dysbiosis? All likely. Throw in as well twenty years of oral birth control use, levothyroxine for twenty-five years, gluten intolerance, an unknown viral infection in my 20s, antibiotics for surgeries to remove a tumour from my spine, and years of sugar and wine cravings. Lovely.

I did put in the work. Some foods, such as gluten and dairy, never returned to my diet. Sugar, even after five years of work, still triggers acne. Chocolate, coffee, and black tea are no-gos, far too stimulating, which leads to lightning strikes of pain in my head. Soy gives me gut pangs, like my bowels are twisting up. I can eat tomatoes but not too many, or I get forehead psoriasis and constipation. White potatoes and pork are okay once in a while in small quantities.

Once you know the signs your body gives you, you will know when you have eaten something by mistake. For example, we were at a dinner party one Friday night. I had contacted the host to let her know my dietary restrictions, and she had worked diligently to create a lovely meal that was gluten- and dairy-free. Saturday morning, I woke up and found it difficult to get my brain going. I could drive all right but found my spatial sense challenged as

I pulled in to park. At the trade show, I found my concentration poor, and it was difficult to engage in social conversation. I could feel my immune system responding to something, as the low-grade fatigue and brain fog were classic signs of food sensitivity response. This lasted into Monday morning when I looked in the mirror and on my lower chin was the typical red rash. When I went to work out, my muscles were sluggish and sore. Riding the cycle on a low level was like trying to pedal through slush. Bowel movements on the third and fourth day became larger and more difficult to pass. On the fourth night after, I had achy, twisting pain in the lower right quadrant of my abdomen.

To overcome the bad effects of gluten, I work with a plan that includes eating what I usually eat. This means following the daily diet tips we went over in the previous chapter and leaving out any other foods to which I'm sensitive. Basically, matcha tea with almond milk, nuts and seeds, lots of greens and lean protein. A little fruit and lots of herbal tea, bone broth, and pure water. Move my body gently for at least thirty minutes a day. Then I add in my daily supplements. In the morning, high-dose probiotic, fish oil, an activated vitamin B complex, curcumin with *Boswellia*, bromelain, and quercetin. A couple of capsules of slippery elm in the afternoon with my tea. At night, a sachet of homeopathic magnesium and 2,000 IU of vitamin D. Through the day, a teaspoon morning and afternoon of a custom-blend tincture with *Astragalus*, *Codonopsis*, *Panax ginseng*, reishi mushroom, and *White atractylodes*. I'll pop one or two homeopathic immune supporters called Mucococcinum through the day as well, as I find this helps my immune system fight anything.

In a day or two—though sometimes it takes about a week—I

start to normalize. It takes up to three weeks before my gut feels totally good.

FOOD REINTRODUCTION

After you get the results of your food sensitivity test, you'll map them onto the daily diet tips from the previous chapter, then adjust the fat and carbs ratios according to your desired weight or insulin regulation requirements. Higher fat (6–8 servings per day), lower carb (45 g per day) for heavier people or those with blood glucose swings. Lower fat (4–6 servings per day), higher carb (75–90 g per day) for stressed-out, thin, or very active individuals. You will avoid the foods that come up high on your test for at least three months, maybe more.

Here's how you will reintroduce foods, one at a time.

Let's call the first one you reintroduce food A. This can be a food you believe will not cause too much of a reaction or one you miss most. Many people will leave the foods they feel they react to strongest until last. Take food A and eat it two to three times a day for two to three days. If you experience a reaction (stomach pain, diarrhea, headache, joint pain, eczema, or skin rash), then stop eating it and avoid it again for a longer period. Wait three to five days for the gut lining to repair itself and then try food B. If food A causes no reaction, assume it is good to continue eating. Wait a day or two, then reintroduce food B. Continue on this way until you identify the foods to which you are sensitive and those from which you just needed a break.

ADDITIONAL LABS THAT MAY BE HELPFUL WITH GUT HEALTH

Other lab tests to consider:

- Thyroid panel: TSH, free T3, T4, reverse T3, TPOs, anti-TG
- Iron panel: ferritin, serum iron, transferrin, TIBC
- Nutrient panel: vitamin Bs, RBC magnesium, copper and zinc, vitamin D
- Leaky gut: urine indican (Obermyer test), serum zonulin, ESR, CRP
- Organic acids for neurotransmitters, hormones, fungal overgrowth

Low thyroid function can contribute to slow-moving stool and constipation. It is one of the first things to check for if you have long-standing constipation (meaning you don't go for days) or dry, difficult-to-pass stools. This is because motility of the gastro-intestinal tract depends on you having enough thyroid hormone. The active thyroid hormone (T3) stimulates the production of mitochondria, our energy powerhouses. If you have any doubts about your thyroid, get it checked. If you have a family history of thyroid issues, don't delay the testing. Continue to monitor this marker. Thyroid can be low due to gluten issues (poor nutrient absorption) or low iron, low selenium, or low iodine intake.

Symptoms of low thyroid function include dry brittle hair, thinning of the hair on the outer eyebrows, white spots on nails, dry brittle nails, dry flaky skin, foggy brain, poor memory, low mood, dry difficult stool, sluggishness of all processes in the body, poor uptake of nutrients, feeling cold, fatigue, weight gain or retention of fluids, migraines, poor wound healing, PMS, heavy periods, low blood sugar, poor sex drive, muscle pain, acne, low blood pressure, insomnia, and infertility.

There are many laboratory tests that may serve as a window into your health. If you'd rather not to do the tests, then try this: work through chapters 1–4. Use the daily diet tips and remove any foods you feel are a problem for you. Regardless, eliminate gluten, dairy, and sugar. Get going with this. You can do it slowly like Jeanie did when she made small changes each time she prepared a meal or snack. Start with awareness, then build in action. Then you can work forward into the next chapters, layering more awareness and further action.

You may feel intimidated by the idea of eliminating your favourite foods from your diet. It might be scary to think there is something creepy swimming around in your gut. That's allowed. Lean into these feelings fully. Then, when you are ready, turn the page to arm yourself with the knowledge you can use to fine-tune your gut reset protocol.

SET YOURSELF FREE

Here's what you'll learn in this chapter:

- Gut reset protocol: evidence-based natural medicine
- Importance of individualized treatment
- Finally, you break through the physical layer of the onion.

"Wherever the art of medicine is loved, there is also a love of humanity."

—HIPPOCRATES

Ah, the chapter you have been waiting for! We'll work really hard here to peel the outer layer of the onion. That's your physical layer. Later, you can peel into the emotional, cognitive, and spiritual layers of healing. In this chapter, you will learn the importance of getting the bad guys out and the good guys in and then cleaning up the mess left behind. There are many ways to climb the mountain.

Steps to gut reset are well known and quite simple.

1. Eliminate (weed)
2. Reinoculate (feed)
3. Repair

ELIMINATE OR WEED: GET THE BAD GUYS OUT

Think of weeding a garden. A weed is an unwanted plant. Dandelions might be great for tea and salads, but not everyone wants them in their flower beds. You pull them up by the roots, or they just come back. You can spray the general area to kill all the plants (like broad-spectrum antibiotics), but that kills both good and bad plants, leaving you with little life (not to mention the toxins in the sprays).

Always cook and store food in glass or stainless steel. Avoid plastics and coated pans.

For (at least) three months, eliminate:

- Unwanted pathogens
- Foods to which you are sensitive
- Caffeine (limit to one cup of tea or coffee if necessary)
- Gluten (perhaps all grains if the damage is severe)
- Dairy
- Sugar
- Remove or at least reduce alcohol to 1–3 servings per week
- Packaged and processed foods
- Unnecessary supplements

Review and be aware of the following medications that may affect the gut, but do not quit any without first consulting your prescribing doctor:

- Antibiotics
- Cancer therapies (I don't recommend weeding while you're on these)
- Antihistamines
- Antidiabetic drugs
- Anti-inflammatory drugs
- Gastrointestinal disorder drugs
- Nonsteroidal anti-inflammatory drugs (NSAIDs)
- Antipsychotic drugs
- Anticoagulants
- Hormones: estrogen, birth control, thyroid hormone

"If you think of this world as a place intended simply for our happiness, you find it quite intolerable: think of it as a place of training and correction, and it's not so bad."

—C. S. LEWIS

Natural remedies can be very strong.

Progress may mean you feel a little worse before you feel better, especially in the first three to five days of the program. This is because of the die-off. What I might consider progress, you might say is terrible! That's because you may feel crummy for the first three to five days of the program. This is because die-off of bad bacteria and fungi can release the toxins they hold. If you have a lot of toxins released at once, it is difficult for your body to process it all. You can feel feverish, nauseous, weak, lightheaded, and have a headache or some muscle aches and pains. This is called a Herxheimer reaction. It is not a reaction to the supplements, but instead a reaction to the toxins being released and cleared. It should last only a couple of days, then you will feel better than before. If it is too strong, then just slow down the supplements. Maybe take them twice per day instead of three times, for example. Then build back up to three times a day.

Be sure to keep your electrolytes up. Ones with *no sugar*! You might like a tri-salts with potassium, sodium, and magnesium to serve your electrolyte needs. This is super helpful. So is an activated B-complex vitamin. The microbes in your gut make a lot of your B vitamins. If your microbiome is out of balance, you may need to supplement with B vitamins until your gut is reset. Also, drink plenty of water. Some herbal teas like nettle and dandelion leaf are very helpful to detox the kidneys. Dandelion root supports liver detoxification. As your body gets rid of the unwanted pathogens, it will need extra help to support its natural daily mechanisms of detoxification. That means, if you can, include about twenty minutes of sunshine, thirty minutes of gentle exercise in some fresh air (maybe in the sunshine!), cleansing vegetable broths and teas, good sleep, and lots of rest. All of these things will help support your body. Once you move through this difficult time, you will find clarity in the mind, energy will rise, and strength will build.

UNIQUE SOLUTIONS FOR EACH INDIVIDUAL

I love plants. When I sit in my room with my cabinet of tinctures, I feel like I am among many friends. They are much wiser than I am and always have something new to teach me. Each one has a personality and behaves differently in different circumstances, like a chameleon. Like people, they bring different things to the table and are richer when they work together as a team. That's why you see so many formulas on the market. What's great for one person may not work for another. Custom blends are amazing because you can get the exact formula that suits your needs at a given time. Tinctures are made by taking plant material, crushing it up, and soaking it in alcohol for a time. Sometimes tinctures are dried, then either stuffed into capsules or pressed, with a binding agent, into tablets. Generally, both the tablet and tincture taste awful and bitter. It is important for the plant medicine to hit your tongue because that is where they start to work. Thus, I prefer the tablet or tincture over the capsule. One funny thing I find with a lot of people is that once their body discovers the action of the plant medicine, it almost craves it. Then the bitterness isn't an obstacle anymore.

Different plants target different body parts. A microbiome comprehensive stool analysis will determine which remedies you should use, how much you should take, when you should take it, and for how long. Purity is essential. Too much can be poisonous. There are studies that say some herbal medicines are toxic. So long as the dose is safe, often it is the impurity of the source that is the issue, not the herb (plant) itself.

Reactions can happen to anyone with anything. Not all supplements are safe for all people. What is mentioned here is not intended to replace individualized medical supervision or advice. It is not a shopping list. It is meant to educate and empower you to have a relevant conversation with your medical provider. Plant (botanical, herbal) medicines are active and can interact with existing prescription medication. Please consult your healthcare provider to determine what product, what dose, and for how long it is safe to take. Special note: not all combos are safe for children or for pregnant or breastfeeding mothers. However, many plant medicines are. I may mention some here and there but always safest to check with your prescribing herbalist or naturopathic doctor.

ENTERIC-COATED ESSENTIAL OILS

There are times when the stomach acid can denature the medicine, and it is better for the medicine to be put in a capsule with an enteric coat (a coating the stomach acid can't break down). Then the medicine can do its work in the small intestine or large intestine. That's the idea anyway.

Enteric-coated caraway, peppermint, thyme, clove, or oregano may all be used with some success to reset bacterial imbalances such as bacterial overgrowth in the small intestine (SIBO). Not all essential oils are safe for internal consumption. A trusted brand properly formulated is a safe bet. Not all combos are safe for children.

Peppermint oil that is coated to release in the small intestine is effective, according to research and clinical experience. Many patients see improvement within two weeks, and one to two months of treatment is often enough. I have used enteric-coated peppermint, caraway, fennel, and clove oil in elderly patients with great success. It is helpful with mild cases of SIBO, irritable bowel syndrome (IBS), and general indigestion. Enteric-coated peppermint oil alone has positive results in children. In one study, 75 percent of forty-two children studied had reduced IBS gut after two weeks of treatment.[80] In a review of how well

---

80   Kline, R. M., Kline, J. J., Di Palma J, & Barbero, G. J. (2001). Enteric-coated, pH-dependent peppermint oil capsules for the treatment of irritable bowel syndrome in children. *The Journal of Pediatrics*, *138*(1), 125–128. https://doi.org/10.1067/mpd.2001.109606

enteric-coated peppermint oil works in adults, significant overall improvement of IBS symptoms and reduction in abdominal pain were observed.[81]

OREGANO OIL

Strong stuff. Be careful. Not too much for too long. It will wipe out many colonies of bacteria, fungus, and viruses on many surfaces. Essential oil of oregano can stop *Candida albicans* and other *Candida* species in their tracks.[82] It's the carvacrol in the oregano oil. Oregano oil taken orally also tames overgrowth of *E. coli* in urinary tract infections[83] and works topically on *Staphylococcus* skin infections.[84]

GARLIC (*ALLIUM SATIVUM*)

Garlic is both anti-inflammatory and antimicrobial. It contains seventeen amino acids, over thirty-three sulfur compounds, eight minerals (germanium, calcium, copper, iron, potassium, magnesium, selenium, and zinc), and the vitamins A, B, and C.[85]

81   Khanna, R., MacDonald, J. K., & Levesque, B. G. (2014). Peppermint oil for the treatment of irritable bowel syndrome: A systematic review and meta-analysis. *Journal of Clinical Gastroenterology*, *48*(6), 505–512. https://doi.org/10.1097/MCG.0b013e3182a88357

82   Pozzatti, P., Scheid, L. A., Spader, T. B., Atayde, M. L., Santurio, J. M., & Alves, S. H. (2008). In vitro activity of essential oils extracted from plants used as spices against fluconazole-resistant and fluconazole-susceptible *Candida spp. Canadian Journal of Microbiology*, *54*(11), 950–956. https://doi.org/10.1139/w08-097

83   Lee, J. H., Kim, Y. G., & Lee, J. (2017). Carvacrol-rich oregano oil and thymol-rich thyme red oil inhibit biofilm formation and the virulence of uropathogenic *Escherichia coli. Journal of Applied Microbiology*, *123*(6), 1420–1428. https://doi.org/10.1111/jam.13602

84   Nostro, A., Roccaro, A. S., Bisignano, G., Marino, A., Cannatelli, M. A., Pizzimenti, F. C., Cioni, P. L., Procopio, F., & Blanco, A. R. (2007). Effects of oregano, carvacrol and thymol on *Staphylococcus aureus* and *Staphylococcus epidermidis* biofilms. *Journal of Medical Microbiology*, *56*(Pt 4), 519–523. https://doi.org/10.1099/jmm.0.46804-0

85   Josling, P. (2007). *Allicin: "The Heart of Garlic."* Welwyn Garden City, UK: Natural Health Holdings.

The antimicrobial effects come about when the clove of garlic is crushed, and two parts of the garlic, alliin and alliinase, combine to make allicin. Allicin breaks down the cell walls of viruses, bacteria, and fungi. Allicin is destroyed by stomach acid, so while it works locally in the mouth for upper respiratory symptoms, it needs to be enteric coated to work farther down the gastrointestinal tract. Enteric-coated garlic extract (allicin) can be more effective than nystatin, an antifungal drug, against pathogenic yeasts, especially the biofilms of *Candida albicans*.[86] Garlic also lowers cholesterol and blood pressure. It is safe long term and often taken for months at a time.

BERBERIS AND GRAPEFRUIT SEED EXTRACT

A formula with grapefruit seed extract, vitamin A, and zinc (Citricidal®) is one of my gut reset go-tos. Typically, I pair this with 500 mg *Berberis aquifolium* in capsule form. You take this with food. Usually, I'll prescribe a six-week rotation of this, followed by another formula blend for four to six weeks.

The formula per dose looks like this: 125 mg Oregon grape extract root, which has 97 percent *Berberis aquifolium*, and one tablet of Citracidal®, which has 10 mg zinc and 435 micrograms vitamin A. The grapefruit seed and pulp extract in Citracidal® provide potent bioflavonoids proven to kill more than 800 bacterial and viral strains, 100 strains of fungus, and a large number of single- and multi-celled parasites. The berberine modifies the microbiome resulting in anti-inflammatory effects that reduce

---

86 Khodavandi, A., Harmal, N. S., Alizadeh, F., Scully, O. J., Sidik, S. M., Othman, F., Sekawi, Z., Ng, K. P., & Chong, P. P. (2011). Comparison between allicin and fluconazole in *Candida albicans* biofilm inhibition and in suppression of HWP1 gene expression. *Phytomedicine*, 19(1), 56–63. https://doi.org/10.1016/j.phymed.2011.08.060

obesity, hyperlipidaemia, diabetes, cancer, and inflammatory disease conditions.[87]

This can be taken with food two or, if you can handle it, three times a day. If the die-off reaction is too much for you, then just do the antimicrobials twice per day. You might be able to build up to three times after a few days. With your third meal of the day or your bedtime snack, take the probiotic. Always take the probiotic and the antimicrobials at least two hours apart. Take probiotics later in the day to give them a chance to work overnight.

Some patients even do a five- and two-day, or four- and three-day split; they take the antimicrobials on weekdays and the probiotics on the weekends. Either routine likely works. I just like the twelve-hour rotation and have had good luck with it. I suggest doing it for four to six weeks, then switching to a botanical product that includes *Juglans nigra* (black walnut hull) for another four to six weeks.

In severe cases, I have gone a little slower. That is, I've done the weed protocol for up to six months. Rotation of the plant medicines is the most rounded approach, and this is best if medically supervised. Concurrent testing of the microbiome is highly recommended during pauses of the protocol.

CAPRYLIC ACID

A natural component of coconut and palm oils, caprylic acid works against *Candida* infections, mastitis (breast milk duct

---

87   Habtemariam, S. (2020). Berberine pharmacology and the gut microbiota: A hidden therapeutic link. *Pharmacological Research*, 155, 104722. https://doi.org/10.1016/j.phrs.2020.104722

infection) due to *E. coli*, and *Staphylococcus*. Start with two tablespoons of coconut oil in your diet per day.

Sometimes I use formulas that pair caprylic acid with clove oil, garlic (allicin), and pau d'arco (*Tabebuia heptaphylla*). These formulas are not always safe for breastfeeding mothers, so check with your medical provider to ensure safety. If it's in a formula, you will see magnesium, zinc, or calcium caprylate. It is best if you take it in morning and evening doses, about ten to fifteen minutes before meals. The formula I use contains 500 mg pau d'arco, 360 mg calcium caprylate, 360 mg magnesium caprylate, 80 mg zinc caprylate, 200 mg garlic with 1 percent allicin, and 70 mg clove bud. There are other, similar formulas on the market.

PAU D'ARCO (*TABEBUIA HEPTAPHYLLA*)

This comes from the bark of a tree in the rainforests of Central and South America. Source it from ethical providers. It works against fungi, bacteria, and viruses. Its natural active chemical components, naphthoquinones, do the work. It can be in a formula or a tea. A couple of cups of the tea a day during the weed protocol is a great idea.

JUGLANS NIGRA

Usually found in a tincture or capsule, black walnut shell, or *Juglans nigra*, is very high in tannins. Tannins are also found in black tea. Think of what this inside of a teapot looks like if it is not washed. A black film, right? Plant tannins can help decrease the inflammation of ulcerative colitis (UC). UC patients don't have the benefit of normal barrier protection.

FEED: GET THE GOOD GUYS IN

Reinoculation can include probiotics, prebiotics, digestive enzymes, hydrochloric acid, and unpasteurized apple cider vinegar. It also may mean adding in any nutrients in which you are insufficient or deficient.

PROBIOTICS

Take probiotics with food or get enteric-coated or spore-based capsules to prevent the probiotics from being denatured in stomach acid.

A maintenance dose for *Lactobacillus* and *Bifidobacterium* blend is typically 10–50 billion per day. *Saccharomyces boulardii* is dosed at 5–10 billion per day. In extreme situations after the reset protocol, I will advise VSL#3 or Genestra's HMF Intensive 500B.

Research on probiotics shows that different strains may be helpful to achieve different results. Keep in mind, however, experts have yet to reach consensus on what a healthy microbiome looks like. This makes it difficult to know which probiotic will translate directly into health benefits. Regardless, I want you to meet a few of the good guys.

A healthy microbiota includes several families of bacteria: 70 percent *Bacteroidetes* and *Firmicutes* and 30 percent from the families

Proteobacteria, Verrucomicrobia, Actinobacteria, Fusobacteria, and *Cyanobacteria.*[88,89] Overall, these bacteria families support one another in community and tend to balance each other out, just like humans living in their communities.

Your microbiome plays an important role in mediating depression and anxiety.[90] *Lactobacillus brevis, Bifidobacterium dentium, Bifidobacterium adolescentis,* and *Bifidobacterium infantis* all produce your major calming neurotransmitter, gamma amino butyric acid (GABA). Low GABA may lead to anxiety, insomnia, irritability, and abdominal pain.[91] *Lactobacillus rhamnosus* acts on GABA receptors. This also has implications for pain management. GABA produced by the intestinal microbiome may one day be used to treat abdominal pain.[92] Supplement with the forementioned probiotics to help restore levels of GABA.

SACCHAROMYCES BOULARDII

Saccharomyces boulardii, or *Sac. B.,* is a type of yeast that helps

88 Lankelma, J. M., Nieuwdorp, M., de Vos, W. M., & Wiersinga, W. J. (2015). The gut microbiota in internal medicine: Implications for health and disease. *The Netherlands Journal of Medicine, 73*(2), 61–68.

89 Qin, J., Li, R., Raes, J., Arumugam, M., Burgdorf, K. S., Manichanh, C., Nielsen, T., Pons, N., Levenez, F., Yamada, T., Mende, D. R., Li, J., Xu, J., Li, S., Li, D., Cao, J., Wang, B., Liang, H., Zheng, H., Xie, Y.,...Wang, J. (2010). A human gut microbial gene catalogue established by metagenomic sequencing. *Nature, 464*(7285), 59–65. https://doi.org/10.1038/nature08821

90 Dhakal, R., Bajpai, V. K., & Baek, K. H. (2012). Production of GABA (γ-aminobutyric acid) by microorganisms: A review. *Brazilian Journal of Microbiology, 43*(4), 1230–1241. https://doi.org/10.1590/S1517-83822012000400001

91 Pokusaeva, K., Johnson, C., Luk, B., Uribe, G., Fu, Y., Oezguen, N., Matsunami, R. K., Lugo, M., Major, A., Mori-Akiyama, Y., Hollister, E. B., Dann, S. M., Shi, X. Z., Engler, D. A., Savidge, T., & Versalovic, J. (2017). GABA-producing *Bifidobacterium dentium* modulates visceral sensitivity in the intestine. *Neurogastroenterology and Motility, 29*(1), e12904. https://doi.org/10.1111/nmo.12904

92 Pokusaeva, K., Johnson, C., Luk, B., Uribe, G., Fu, Y., Oezguen, N., Matsunami, R. K., Lugo, M., Major, A., Mori-Akiyama, Y., Hollister, E. B., Dann, S. M., Shi, X. Z., Engler, D. A., Savidge, T., & Versalovic, J. (2017). GABA-producing *Bifidobacterium dentium* modulates visceral sensitivity in the intestine. *Neurogastroenterology and Motility, 29*(1), e12904. https://doi.org/10.1111/nmo.12904

crowd out *Candida albicans* and tame the *Clostridium* species. It is used to relieve traveller's diarrhea and hospital-borne diarrhea from *C. difficile* (*Clostridium* family). *Sac. B.* shows promise of being able to reduce intestinal cell inflammation and help heal the damage gluten does to the gut.[93] It does this by promoting IgA production. When 250 mg of *Sac. B.* is administered three meals a day with the drug mesalazine for four weeks, seventeen out of twenty-four patients achieve endoscopic remission. This could be the very means it helps reduce stool frequency in those suffering from colitis.[94]

Although *Sac. B.* is helpful, you don't want to take too much for too long because it could backfire, and you could end up with other yeast-related health issues. How long is too long? It depends on the individual, but I'd say it's generally safe to supplement for six months.

LACTOBACILLUS SPECIES

Lactobacillus species have a number of different strains, which can help in various ways.

L. ACIDOPHILUS

Acidophilus preserves a lot of food. You will find it in naturally fermented yogurt. In the gut, it is one of the best strains to produce

---

93 Papista, C., Gerakopoulos, V., Kourelis, A., Sounidaki, M., Kontana, A., Berthelot, L., Moura, I. C., Monteiro, R. C., & Yiangou, M. (2012). Gluten induces coeliac-like disease in sensitised mice involving IgA, CD71 and transglutaminase 2 interactions that are prevented by probiotics. *Laboratory Investigation, 92*(4), 625-635. https://doi.org/10.1038/labinvest.2012.13

94 Guslandi, M., Giollo, P., & Testoni, P. A. (2003). A pilot trial of *Saccharomyces boulardii* in ulcerative colitis. *European Journal of Gastroenterology & Hepatology, 15*(6), 697-698. https://doi.org/10.1097/00042737-200306000-00017

those helpful short-chain fatty acids (SCFAs) and protects from the harmful impact of viruses and infectious bacteria. It also aids in vaginal infection (yeast, vaginosis) healing. Save introducing yogurt into the diet until the weed protocol is complete.

L. PLANTARUM

Another food preservative, *L. plantarum*, is what naturally ferments milk to kefir, cabbage to sauerkraut, and other vegetables to kimchi. It preserves intestinal lining (mucosa) and inhibits pathogenic bacteria and opportunistic yeast overgrowth. It can survive some broad-spectrum antibiotics. *L. plantarum* can help prevent and treat IBS, inflammatory bowel disease,[95] cancer, metabolic syndromes, dyslipidemia, hypercholesteremia, obesity, diabetes, and brain conditions including psychological disorders.[96] Save introducing fermented foods into the diet until after the weed protocol is complete.

L. CASEI

This species is found in raw milk, hard-cooked, long-ripened cheese such as Parmigiano-Reggiano and Grana Padano.[97] Medicinally, it is used to treat intestinal infections by improving your immunity against bacteria and viruses. You may want to avoid this one if you tend to have high histamine or get hives from foods or environmental sensitivities.

---

95 Le, B., & Yang, S. H. (2018). Efficacy of *Lactobacillus plantarum* in prevention of inflammatory bowel disease. *Toxicology Reports, 5*, 314-317. https://doi.org/10.1016/j.toxrep.2018.02.007

96 Liu, Y. W., Liong, M. T., & Tsai, Y. C. (2018). New perspectives of *Lactobacillus plantarum* as a probiotic: The gut-heart-brain axis. *Journal of Microbiology, 56*(9), 601-613. https://doi.org/10.1007/s12275-018-8079-2

97 Bottari, B., Levante, A., Neviani, E., & Gatti, M. (2018). How the fewest become the greatest: *L. casei*'s impact on long ripened cheeses. *Frontiers in Microbiology, 9*, 2866. https://doi.org/10.3389/fmicb.2018.02866

L. SALIVARIUS

L. salivarius suppresses the growth of pathogenic (harmful) bacteria and reduces gas. It can treat acne vulgaris[98] and improve oral hygiene by reducing bad breath and cavities.[99] The *L. salivarius PS7* shows promise for the prevention of ear infections in infants and children.[100] The MG242 version may be used to treat or prevent vaginal candidiasis.[101]

L. PARACASEI

It is a common inhabitant of the mucosal lining of healthy individuals, contributing to favourable intestinal acidity for great health.

L. REUTERI

L. reuteri helps breastfed babies who experience infantile colic.[102] It is also known to fight infections and strengthen the immune response.

---

98 Deidda, F., Amoruso, A., Nicola, S., Graziano, T., Pane, M., & Mogna, L. (2018). New approach in acne therapy: A specific bacteriocin activity and a targeted anti IL-8 property in just 1 probiotic strain, the *L. salivarius* LS03. *Journal of Clinical Gastroenterology, 52*(Suppl 1), S78–S81. https://doi.org/10.1097/MCG.0000000000001053

99 Higuchi, T., Suzuki, N., Nakaya, S., Omagari, S., Yoneda, M., Hanioka, T., & Hirofuji, T. (2019). Effects of *Lactobacillus salivarius* WB21 combined with green tea catechins on dental caries, periodontitis, and oral malodor. *Archives of Oral Biology, 98*, 243–247. https://doi.org/10.1016/j.archoralbio.2018.11.027

100 Cárdenas, N., Martín, V., Arroyo, R., et al. (2019). Prevention of recurrent acute otitis media in children through the use of *Lactobacillus salivarius* PS7, a target-specific probiotic strain. *Nutrients, 11*(2), 376. https://doi.org/10.3390/nu11020376

101 Kang, C. H., Han, S. H., Kim, Y., Paek, N. S., & So, J. S. (2018). In vitro probiotic properties of *Lactobacillus salivarius* MG242 isolated from human vagina. *Probiotics and Antimicrobial Proteins, 10*(2), 343–349. https://doi.org/10.1007/s12602-017-9323-5

102 Anabrees, J., Indrio, F., Paes, B., & AlFaleh, K. (2013). Probiotics for infantile colic: A systematic review. *BMC Pediatrics, 13*, 186. https://doi.org/10.1186/1471-2431-13-186

L. RHAMNOSUS

L. rhamnosus GR-1 and *L. reuteri* RC-14 show strong antifungal activity against vulvovaginal candidiasis (*Candida glabrata*[103]).

BIFIDOBACTERIUM SPECIES

In addition to all the *Lactobacillus* species, *Bifidobacterium* is one of the more stable and dominant groups within your microbiome. It is part of the *Actinobacteria* family. Why is it so strong? It feeds off many kinds of carbohydrates and has superior energy output.[104] *Bifidobacterium* alleviates infection, produces lactic acid (lowers pH of the intestine), improves tolerance to lactose, lowers cholesterol,[105] and helps alleviate diarrhea and constipation.[106] It also maintains remission in ulcerative colitis.[107] Low levels of *Bifidobacterium* are associated with clinical depression in those with IBS. A strict vegetarian diet may help restore deficiencies.

103 Chew, S. Y., Cheah, Y. K., Seow, H. F., Sandai, D., & Than, L. T. (2015). Probiotic *Lactobacillus rhamnosus* GR-1 and *Lactobacillus reuteri* RC-14 exhibit strong antifungal effects against vulvovaginal candidiasis-causing *Candida glabrata* isolates. *Journal of Applied Microbiology, 118*(5), 1180–1190. https://doi.org/10.1111/jam.12772

104 Odamaki, T., Bottacini, F., Kato, K., Mitsuyama, E., Yoshida, K., Horigome, A., Xiao, J. Z., & van Sinderen, D. (2018). Genomic diversity and distribution of *Bifidobacterium longum* subsp. *longum* across the human lifespan. *Scientific Reports, 8*(1), 85. https://doi.org/10.1038/s41598-017-18391-x

105 Kriaa, A., Bourgin, M., Potiron, A., Mkaouar, H., Jablaoui, A., Gérard, P., Maguin, E., & Rhimi, M. (2019). Microbial impact on cholesterol and bile acid metabolism: Current status and future prospects. *Journal of Lipid Research, 60*(2), 323-332. https://doi.org/10.1194/jlr.R088989

106 Ibarra, A., Latreille-Barbier, M., Donazzolo, Y., Pelletier, X., & Ouwehand, A. C. (2018). Effects of 28-day *Bifidobacterium animalis* subsp. *lactis* HN019 supplementation on colonic transit time and gastrointestinal symptoms in adults with functional constipation: A double-blind, randomized, placebo-controlled, and dose-ranging trial. *Gut Microbes, 9*(3), 236-251. https://doi.org/10.1080/19490976.2017.1412908

107 Zuo, L., Yuan, K. T., Yu, L., Meng, Q. H., Chung, P. C., & Yang, D. H. (2014). *Bifidobacterium infantis* attenuates colitis by regulating T cell subset responses. *World Journal of Gastroenterology, 20*(48), 18316–18329. https://doi.org/10.3748/wjg.v20.i48.18316

PREBIOTICS

Initially, you will want to skip the prebiotics. If you don't have enough good guys down there and/or have too many bad guys, then the prebiotics will only worsen your gas, pain, bloat, and fatigue.

Be mindful when you introduce any prebiotics into your routine, and when you do, start low and slow.

Fructans such as fructo-oligosaccharides (FOS) and inulin, as well as galactins such as galacto-oligosaccharides (GOS), are the most studied prebiotics. They are found in leek, onion, garlic, artichoke, chicory, asparagus, banana, rye, and corn. Fibres in starchy vegetables will help, too. With a healthy microbiome, you can set a goal to consume 3–11 g of natural prebiotics per day. If the microbiome is imbalanced, you may want to restrict prebiotics until you have healthy flora. This is what the FODMAPs diet is all about.

According to expert consensus, prebiotics must meet three criteria:[108]

1. Be resistant to digestion in the stomach and upper intestine
2. Be fermentable by the gut microbiota
3. Specifically stimulate the growth and/or activity of intestinal bacteria beneficial to our health

---

108 Gibson, G. R., Hutkins, R., Sanders, M. E., Prescott, S. L., Reimer, R. A., Salminen, S. J., Scott, K., Stanton, C., Swanson, K. S., Cani, P. D., Verbeke, K., & Reid, G. (2017). Expert consensus document: The International Scientific Association for Probiotics and Prebiotics (ISAPP) consensus statement on the definition and scope of prebiotics. *Nature Reviews: Gastroenterology & Hepatology, 14*(8), 491–502. https://doi.org/10.1038/nrgastro.2017.75

Inulin is an important prebiotic to nurture a healthy microbiome. Chicory root contains the highest amount of inulin. It is often added to processed foods for flavour and fibre and to probiotics as a prebiotic. You can consume it directly as the root as a coffee substitute and the leaves can be used for bitter greens in a salad.

Other remedies worth mentioning are ones that both feed and help heal the gut: herbal prebiotics, which include slippery elm (*Ulmus rubra*), marshmallow root extract (*Althea off.*), and edible aloe vera gel concentrate.

Green tea (up to six cups per day or 300 mg of green tea catechins) can also raise levels of *Bifido* and *Lactobacillus* bacteria while lowering levels of *Enterobacteriaceae, Bacteridacea*, and *Eubacteria*.[109] Thus, green tea boosts the immune system. Besides cleansing and detoxifying vital organs, it also lowers cholesterol, blood pressure, and blood sugar levels. It helps prevent obesity by modifying the microbiome.[110] A powerful antioxidant, green tea helps prevent and reduce cancer, arterial sclerosis, strokes, and heart disease. Just watch the caffeine levels. Green tea caffeine is a slower burn, so it doesn't spike like coffee, chocolate, or other teas. Depending on your genetic makeup, it still may make you jittery and affect your sleep.

Acacia gum benefits the aging microbiome. It increases *Bifidobacterium* and helps with constipation. Likewise, gluten-free SunFibre® is helpful, as are other brands that contain partially

---

109 Hara, Y. (1997). Influence of tea catechins on the digestive tract. *Journal of Cellular Biochemistry: Supplement, 27*, 52–58.

110 Zhu, J., Cai, R., Tan, Y., Wu, X., Wen, Q., Liu, Z., Ouyang, S. H., Yin, Z., & Yang, H. (2020). Preventive consumption of green tea modifies the gut microbiota and provides persistent protection from high-fat diet-induced obesity. *Journal of Functional Foods, 64*, 103621. https://doi.org/10.1016/j.jff.2019.103621

hydrolyzed guar gum (PHGG). You can also try a quarter teaspoon potato starch, so long as you are not sensitive to the nightshade family. Just watch out for those products that are labelled *Solanum tuberosum* and charge $30–$40 for a small packet. This is an unnecessary expenditure. If you prefer, you can even just eat a few tablespoons of cooked and cooled rice or potatoes a few days a week, as these foods contain the resistant starch naturally.

If you focus on prebiotics for at least six weeks, while also taking probiotics, you will get the flora flourishing. For people with chronic diseases, such as autoimmune conditions, the entire feed protocol will require months of ongoing therapy.

DIGESTIVE AIDS

HYDROCHLORIC ACID AND UNPASTEURIZED APPLE CIDER VINEGAR

The stomach acid barrier is an important line of defence in the maintenance of a healthy gut flora. As you just read above, adequate stomach acid is also required to stimulate digestive enzymes. I like unpasteurized organic apple cider vinegar (ACV).

Get a shot glass, measure two tablespoons of ACV, and mark the line. You can take this right before, during, or after a meal. Initially, I recommend taking it at every large meal for two weeks. There will come a point at which you can't take it anymore and you'll likely gag at the feeling of it in your mouth. It may feel like that at first, but give it a try for a few days. If it still feels like that, then you likely don't need the ACV. If you've done it for a week or two and the gag happens, that's when you're done with the daily dose. Then you may just take it once in a while when you feel like food is sitting around too long in the stomach. For now, take a dose of the ACV and see how it goes. Always rinse your mouth immediately after the ACV. Otherwise, it will do a number on your tooth enamel.

DIGESTIVE ENZYMES

If the pancreas isn't working well (and there are many reasons why it might not be) or its ducts are blocked, enzymes won't reach their destination. Chronic untreated celiac or inflammatory bowel disease (IBD) and loss of integrity of the small intestinal border prevent proper enzyme function and stop nutrients from being absorbed. While executing the gut protocol, you may wish to include digestive enzymes to help stimulate progress and boost your vitality. Consider starting with ACV to boost acid in the stomach (only if there are no stomach or small intestine ulcers). If, after two weeks, the ACV doesn't help with the digestion process, I may add in three to six month's use of digestive enzymes with larger meals. The goal is to not have so many supplements, but sometimes short-term supplementation can really make a difference.

GENTIAN

I can't leave the digestive stimulation train of thought without mentioning *Gentian lutea*, a very bitter herb and powerful stimulant for digestion. Just a few drops of this before a meal can help ignite the digestive fire!

MOLYBDENUM

Candida is a yeast-producing alcohol, and thus it produces acetaldehydes from the sugars ingested. It takes a lot for your body's enzymes to detox excess acetaldehydes. This leads to multiple chemical sensitivity, especially fragrances. Molybdenum supports acetaldehyde metabolism and helps with sulfite sensitivity (converts sulfites to sulfates). Molybdenum supports acetaldehyde metabolism and helps those with a food or chemical sulfite sensitivity as it detoxifies it into sulfate for excretion. For those with issues with the brassica family of vegetables, garlic, or onions, which are high in sulfur compounds, 150 mg twice per day of molybdenum for a couple of months along with their *Candida* cleanse might be all they need to overcome their sensitivity. I'd be more cautious about use for sensitivity to sulfa drugs, as those reactions can be a little more severe.

REPAIR

The final step for the gut reset is repair.

How you approach this step depends on the state of your health and your preferences when it comes to tinctures, supplements, teas, and food. Sure, there are plenty of remedies out there, but I like to keep it simple and have found a few things to choose from, and they work. There are a few vitamins and minerals that are essential to gut healing. You can start these at any time during the protocol and continue for some time after. Rotation of the repair foods and supplements can help diversify and feed your hungry microbiome.

Foods that are high in antioxidants will help reduce inflammation and improve conditions for those suffering from IBD. Green tea, slippery elm tea, pomegranate and apples, bitter melon, blueberries, bilberries, ginger, and turmeric can all be helpful hands in the kitchen.

VITAMIN A

Vitamin A can improve immune actions against parasitic infections.[111] It helps maintain membranes and aids in immune function, which contributes to microbiome development.[112]

VITAMIN D

Vitamin D is critical to all the cells in the body, especially those that turn over frequently. The lining of the gastrointestinal tract renews every three to five days. Vitamin D is needed to keep the cells linked together and promotes a balanced microbiome.[113] Many people with autoimmune conditions have low levels of vitamin D. We also see trends of autoimmune disease following breaks in the gut barrier (leaky gut). If vitamin D isn't there to hold the cells together, things in the gut leak out into the body. The immune system in the bloodstream attacks the foreign par-

111 Lima, A. A., Soares, A. M., Lima, N. L., et al. (2010). Effects of vitamin A supplementation on intestinal barrier function, growth, total parasitic, and specific *Giardia* spp. infections in Brazilian children: A prospective randomized, double-blind, placebo-controlled trial. *Journal of Pediatric Gastroenterology and Nutrition, 50*(3), 309-315. https://doi.org/10.1097/MPG.0b013e3181a96489

112 Huda, M. N., Ahmad, S. M., Kalanetra, K. M., Taft, D. H., Alam, M. J., Khanam, A., Raqib, R., Underwood, M. A., Mills, D. A., & Stephensen, C. B. (2019). Neonatal vitamin A supplementation and vitamin A status are associated with gut microbiome composition in Bangladeshi infants in early infancy and at 2 years of age. *The Journal of Nutrition, 149*(6), 1075-1088. https://doi.org/10.1093/jn/nxz034

113 Gominak, S. C. (2016). Vitamin D deficiency changes the intestinal microbiome reducing B vitamin production in the gut. The resulting lack of pantothenic acid adversely affects the immune system, producing a "pro-inflammatory" state associated with atherosclerosis and autoimmunity. *Medical Hypotheses, 94*, 103-107. https://doi.org/10.1016/j.mehy.2016.07.007

ticles and launches an inflammatory attack. Chronic attacks lead to chronic inflammation, which leads to parts of the body getting attacked in the process. That's autoimmune. It is important to get vitamin D levels checked, then dose according to the amount you will need for the time you need it to achieve, and then maintain healthy recommended levels.

ZINC

Zinc heals the gut lining, helps your immune system, and controls inflammation. Zinc is found in red meat, some shellfish, legumes, pumpkin seeds, fortified cereals, and whole grains.[114] Since cereals and whole grains have their own issues, eat the other stuff! Or take a supplement. Overall, zinc supplementation can lower inflammation and reduce infection occurrence.[115,116] Careful, though: more is not always better. Long-term or excessive supplementation of zinc may disrupt copper balance. I'll typically dose it for the duration of the gut reset protocol, then stop. Many of the formulas I use with patients include zinc, so additional supplementation is not always necessary. On its own, zinc can be used to repair after a gluten exposure or to halt the onset of a cold or upper respiratory tract infection.

---

114   Gammoh, N. Z., & Rink, L. (2017). Zinc in infection and inflammation. *Nutrients*, 9(6), 624. https://doi. org/10.3390/nu9060624

115   Prasad, A. S., Beck, F. W., Bao, B., Fitzgerald, J. T., Snell, D. C., Steinberg, J. D., & Cardozo, L. J. (2007). Zinc supplementation decreases incidence of infections in the elderly: Effect of zinc on generation of cytokines and oxidative stress. *The American Journal of Clinical Nutrition*, 85(3), 837–844. https://doi.org/10.1093/ ajcn/85.3.837

116   Besecker, B. Y., Exline, M. C., Hollyfield, J., Phillips, G., Disilvestro, R. A., Wewers, M. D., & Knoell, D. L. (2011). A comparison of zinc metabolism, inflammation, and disease severity in critically ill infected and noninfected adults early after intensive care unit admission. *The American Journal of Clinical Nutrition*, 93(6), 1356–1364. https://doi.org/10.3945/ajcn.110.008417

MAGNESIUM

It's responsible for over 300 different transactions in the body, and over 50 percent of the population is deficient. Magnesium deficiency is linked to a number of chronic diseases, including chronic inflammation, atherosclerosis, hypertension, cardiac arrhythmias, stroke, alterations in lipid metabolism, insulin resistance, metabolic syndrome, type 2 diabetes mellitus, and osteoporosis, as well as anxiety, depression, and other neuropsychiatric disorders.[117]

Magnesium occurs naturally in dark leafy greens, nuts, and seeds. With the increased use of fertilizers and intake of processed foods, people are getting less naturally occurring magnesium. To boost magnesium content of garden-grown leafies, add two tablespoons of Epsom salts (magnesium sulfide) to a gallon of their water once a month.

Magnesium loves to bind to stuff, so you will find it in formulas like magnesium oxide, magnesium bisglycinate, and magnesium citrate, to name a few. It also binds with some medications, so always take it an hour or two away from prescription meds. You can take it throughout the day, but I like it best before bed because it helps your muscles relax and relieves anxiety. The maximum recommended daily intake is 600 mg, usually 300 mg in the morning and 300 mg in the evening. I've prescribed lower doses like 300 mg/day and then upped the dose if muscle pains, period cramps, or headaches occurred. But I've also found doing high levels initially, then lowering the amounts to a maintenance dose works well. It depends on the individual.

---

117 Gröber, U., Schmidt, J., & Kisters, K. (2015). Magnesium in prevention and therapy. *Nutrients, 7*(9), 8199–8226. https://doi.org/10.3390/nu7095388

Magnesium is primarily absorbed in the small intestine. If you have a compromised intestinal lining, as with other nutrients, you will struggle to get enough magnesium per day.

- Magnesium oxide is best for treating constipation because most of it stays in the intestines. For severe constipation, you will need to take a high dose for the first 24–48 hours, somewhere around 3,000–4,000 mg (total amount for the day) in divided doses. This means if you have the 400 mg capsules, you need to take eight to ten, spaced evenly throughout the day. Then for your maintenance dose (so you never get constipated again), you take somewhere near 500–700 mg a day, preferably before bed.
- Milk of magnesia is also an effective treatment for constipation, especially during pregnancy. This is a fast-acting magnesium in liquid form, the most recommended constipation cure by doctors. For dosages and advice, simply follow the directions on the bottle.
- Magnesium citrate works extremely well against constipation. If you have anxiety and are constipated, choose this one! You can buy this in either a liquid or powdered form. The dose depends on your bowel tolerance. Diarrhea is the result of too much!
- Magnesium bisglycinate is the one to take for anxiety and body aches and pains. It's the easiest to absorb. Up to 600 mg per day on an ongoing basis is safe. You may not need that much.
- Magnesium threonate has the ability to pass through the blood-brain barrier. This one is best for migraine prevention.

DR. GODFREY'S GUT-HEALING FORMULA

Take this gut-healing remedy on an empty stomach so the goods can get where they need to go: *Althea officianalis* (marshmallow root), *Mentha* (peppermint), *Matricaria* (chamomile), and *Filipendula* mixed in equal parts. Take one teaspoon two to three times a day. It's really quite lovely. Get an herbalist or a qualified naturopathic doctor to put this together for you. I got the formula from our beloved Dr. Godfrey, rest his soul. I use it in honour of him, and he does good work. It is an anti-inflammatory formula that promotes the health of cells in the gut lining. I'll do a round (go through a 250 mL bottle) of this if I have an unexpected gluten encounter.

ULMUS RUBRA (SLIPPERY ELM)

Another great remedy to heal the gut and soothe the distress in the lining is *Ulmus rubra* (slippery elm). Even if you have FODMAP sensitivities, you might find this is a good tool without issue. It comes in capsule or as a powder to make tea. Love this remedy.

DGL

This one is popular in gastro-reflux (GERD/heartburn) because it can soothe the esophagus without affecting blood pressure. Deglycerinated licorice (DGL) in a chewable capsule will help heal the mucosal lining as well.

COLOSTRUM

Colostrum, the early let-down product of breast milk, serves the immunity and, ultimately, gut function. It is speculated that those who were not breastfed are set back in their early development. Bovine (cow) colostrum supplementation improves flora and the gut lining. One study took sixteen athletes with leaky gut and fed them 500 mg colostrum twice daily for twenty days.[118] Seventy-five percent on colostrum (vs. plain whey powder) had improved intestinal permeability status. Colostrum also improves autoimmunity and allergies.[119]

L-GLUTAMINE

I don't recommend it. True, L-glutamine feeds enterocytes (gut-lining cells). It also feeds *Candida* and inflammation, which you likely have if you are doing the gut reset. L-glutamine also comes naturally in your diet if you include foods such as beef, skim milk, tofu, egg, corn, and rice. With all that said, you may or may not benefit from supplementation. In general, if you're a healthy individual with a balanced diet, glutamine supplementation won't really change your state of health. You may consider supplementation if your stores of glutamine are low and if you are an elite athlete; immune-suppressed; experiencing major and/or critical illness, sepsis, trauma, and postsurgery circumstances; or suffer from chronic weakness and several nutritional limitations. A typical supplemental dose is 20–35 g/24 hours.[120]

---

118 Hałasa, M., Maciejewska, D., Baśkiewicz-Hałasa, M., Machaliński, B., Safranow, K., & Stachowska, E. (2017). Oral supplementation with bovine colostrum decreases intestinal permeability and stool concentrations of zonulin in athletes. *Nutrients*, 9(4), 370. https://doi.org/10.3390/nu9040370

119 Boldogh, I., Aguilera-Aguirre, L., Bacsi, A., Choudhury, B. K., Saavedra-Molina, A., & Kruzel, M. (2008). Colostrinin decreases hypersensitivity and allergic responses to common allergens. *International Archives of Allergy and Immunology*, 146(4), 298-306. https://doi.org/10.1159/000121464

120 Cruzat, V., Macedo Rogero, M., Noel Keane, K., Curi, R., & Newsholme, P. (2018). Glutamine: Metabolism and immune function, supplementation and clinical translation. *Nutrients*, 10(11), 1564. https://doi.org/10.3390/nu10111564

TWO BAKED APPLES A DAY

The pectin that gets released when apples are cooked with their skins is very healing to the gut. I smell them cooking in my oven right now. Yum. Pectin protects you from the toxins bad bacteria release (LPS). It increases intestinal alkaline phosphatase (IAP) levels. That helps with cholesterol and fat management. Apple pectin protects you from leaky gut, prevents weight gain, and reduces inflammation.[121] Buy organic apples if you can. Always wash your produce well. In addition to water, I like to use vinegar or lemon juice or grapefruit seed extract. Or a sink full of salted water. My favorite way to prepare the apples is to use one of those apple coring kitchen tools, then lay the apples in a pan. Put enough water to touch the bottoms of the apples. Maybe a quarter of an inch. Sprinkle cinnamon on them and bake in the oven. I often put them in alongside the chicken or vegetables or whatever else happens to be cooking at the time. On their own, they take about forty-five minutes at 350°F, but time depends on the type of apple and how ripe they are. When they are soft and you can poke them easily with a fork, they are done. If you like them a little crispy and dry, don't put so much water on them. If you prefer them juicy and soft, add more water. I'll even throw the apples alongside the roast chicken with carrots, potatoes, celery, and cauliflower. Put some water—maybe half an inch—with the chicken and cover the pan to keep the moisture locked in. Apple pectin is a simple and tasty way to increase your gut's healing power. See? An apple a day can really help keep the doctor away!

121 Jiang, T., Gao, X., Wu, C., Tian, F., Lei, Q., Bi, J., Xie, B., Wang, H. Y., Chen, S., & Wang, X. (2016). Apple-derived pectin modulates gut microbiota, improves gut barrier function, and attenuates metabolic endotoxemia in rats with diet-induced obesity. *Nutrients, 8*(3), 126. https://doi.org/10.3390/nu8030126

BROTH AND COLLAGEN POWDER

Bone broth is lovely, and so is most organic collagen powder, which will provide nutrients to build tissue. Buy organic or responsibly raised sources, or wild game you hunt, so you are consuming the cleanest source. Your hair, skin, and nails will thank you once nutrients start absorbing again. A cup of broth or collagen added to your hot beverage in the morning works great if you take it at least three days a week. If you really need gut protection, take up to four cups a day for four weeks. But if you only get it in once in a while, it will still be helpful. The protein and the gelatin tannate help reduce the effects of inflammatory toxins in the gut. The gelatin in the broth mimics the protective slimy layer your gut might not be making when it is damaged. Under the gelatin's protective soft coat, the intestinal lining can repair. Cellular repair also requires protein, which bone broth gives you. Other forms of protein are helpful, too. BCAAs, or branched-chain amino acids (leucine, isoleucine, and valine), play an important role in gut health, glucose balance, anti-obesity, nutritional status, immunity, and disease.[122] You will find these in foods like beef, chicken, fish, eggs, baked beans, lima beans, chickpeas, lentils, brown rice, almonds, brazil nuts, cashews, and pumpkin seeds. If you like, you can also take a supplement. If you are sensitive to any of these foods, don't eat them.

OLIVE LEAF OIL

Olive oil, produced by crushing the olive fruit, is known for its many heart health benefits. Its plant powers include biophenols that are antioxidant, anti-inflammatory, and cardioprotective,

---

122 Nie, C., He, T., Zhang, W., Zhang, G., & Ma, X. (2018). Branched chain amino acids: Beyond nutrition metabolism. *International Journal of Molecular Sciences, 19*(4), 954. https://doi.org/10.3390/ijms19040954

and lower cholesterol and blood sugar. Did you know that the essential oil gathered from olive *leaves* and *branches* is also helpful for gut inflammation?[123] A much stronger extract than the fruit of the olive, oil from leaves and branches contains 80 percent oleuropein, a biophenol. Within twenty-four hours, it can relieve inflammation in the intestines. This may be something to consider for outbreaks in ulcerative colitis and Crohn's disease.[124] Although not as strong, liberal amounts of regular olive oil are helpful, too.

FISH OIL

Fish oil reduces inflammation body-wide, and in the gut, it can help modulate the balance of bacteria, reduce the risk of IBD and provide and maintain remission of ulcerative colitis.[125] Omega-3s found in fish oil are essential fatty acids, which can also lower cholesterol, regulate insulin,[126] and reduce the risk of many cancers. For various periods of time, 1,200 mg to 20 g a day can be supplemented.

---

123 Larussa, T., Imeneo, M., & Luzza, F. (2019). Olive tree biophenols in inflammatory bowel disease: When bitter is better. *International Journal of molecular Sciences, 20*(6), 1390. https://doi.org/10.3390/ijms20061390

124 Vezza, T., Algieri, F., Rodríguez-Nogales, A., Garrido-Mesa, J., Utrilla, M. P., Talhaoui, N., Gómez-Caravaca, A. M., Segura-Carretero, A., Rodríguez-Cabezas, M. E., Monteleone, G., & Gálvez, J. (2017). Immunomodulatory properties of *Olea europaea* leaf extract in intestinal inflammation. *Molecular Nutrition & Food Research, 61*(10), 10.1002/mnfr.201601066. https://doi.org/10.1002/mnfr.201601066

125 Marton, L. T., Goulart, R. A., Carvalho, A., & Barbalho, S. M. (2019). Omega fatty acids and inflammatory bowel diseases: An overview. *International Journal of Molecular Sciences, 20*(19), 4851. https://doi.org/10.3390/ijms20194851

126 Khatib, S. A., Rossi, E. L., Bowers, L. W., & Hursting, S. D. (2016). Reducing the burden of obesity-associated cancers with anti-inflammatory long-chain omega-3 polyunsaturated fatty acids. *Prostaglandins & Other Lipid Mediators, 125*, 100–107. https://doi.org/10.1016/j.prostaglandins.2016.07.011

FRANKINCENSE (*BOSWELLIA SERRATA*)

Yes, this is the same coveted resin the kings brought Baby Jesus. *Boswellia serrata*, or oleo-gum resin, is a traditional Ayurvedic remedy for inflammatory diseases. It's also known as Salai Guggal, Indian olibanu, or Indian frankincense.[127] It's been found that 350–500 mg, three times a day for at least three months helps put colitis into remission in 82 percent of patients.[128] It puts a brake on motility in the gut to prevent diarrhea. It also has many anti-inflammatory properties.

MARY'S STORY

Mary came to me with colitis, diagnosed after the birth of her first child. She recalls no problems whatsoever before birth. Pregnancy itself is an inflammatory state. In the first trimester, when the egg is implanted into the uterus, and again as the body prepares for delivery, there are increased factors of inflammation. Mary aggravated what must have been an already existing immune-mediated inflammation, and the additional inflammation was the tipping point.

In her experience, Mary finds drugs too harsh and prefers to use food alone as her remedy. She can eat some nuts but finds if she eats too many, it sets her off. She also finds that stress can worsen her symptoms. She eats no gluten, dairy, or sugar and finds this most helpful for her condition. Mary finds slippery elm tea can

127 Catanzaro, D., Rancan, S., Orso, G., Dall'Acqua, S., Brun, P., Giron, M. C., Carrara, M., Castagliuolo, I., Ragazzi, E., Caparrotta, L., & Montopoli, M. (2015). *Boswellia serrata* preserves intestinal epithelial barrier from oxidative and inflammatory damage. *PloS One*, *10*(5), e0125375. https://doi.org/10.1371/journal.pone.0125375

128 Gupta, I., Parihar, A., Malhotra, P., Singh, G. B., Lüdtke, R., Safayhi, H., & Ammon, H. P. (1997). Effects of *Boswellia serrata* gum resin in patients with ulcerative colitis. *European Journal of Medical Research*, *2*(1), 37–43.

calm the bowels and includes it in her diet when she experiences a flare. She begins using *Boswellia* to help calm the inflammation and put her colitis into remission. It takes a while to come around to normal, but she feels she can manage best this way. There is no right or wrong. As long as Mary is pleased with her management and she does not put her long-term health at risk, there should be no reason for her to do anything different. She understands if things get out of control, she has options and knows them well.

CURCUMIN

Talk about a powerhouse! Curcumin is a yellow pigment found in turmeric root (*Curcuma longa*). It has anti-inflammatory, antioxidant, anticancer, antiproliferative, antifungal, and antimicrobial activity. It is known as an anti-*H. pylori* agent along with its help in IBS, dyspepsia, gastric ulcer, pancreatitis, ulcerative colitis, gastrointestinal cancers, and other gastrointestinal diseases.[129] The body doesn't absorb curcumin very well, which is a problem if you want body-wide benefits. Regardless, it can help heal the gut. If it stays in the gut, it's going to help the cells there. Yes, turmeric in the diet can help the cells in the gut. There are a few patented formulated versions of it that claim to make it more absorbable. Look for well-recognized, quality brands. The amount to take will vary based on how well you can absorb it. That's why it's best to check with your medical provider for individual advice based on the product selected. Longvida® formulas are coated in fats to help you absorb them better. Even a two-week treatment

---

129 Sarkar, A., De, R., & Mukhopadhyay, A. K. (2016). Curcumin as a potential therapeutic candidate for *Helicobacter pylori* associated diseases. *World Journal of Gastroenterology, 22*(9), 2736–2748. https://doi.org/10.3748/wjg.v22.i9.2736

can show benefits. Up to three months of treatment will improve ulcers in almost 76 percent of patients.[130]

CHAGA JAVA

Mushroom tea is a bitter, earthy taste. Often, they sell it in packs with coffee to help people cut down on their caffeine. One of my herbal suppliers has packaged chaga mushroom extract with roasted dandelion and chicory root. Nice! The inulin in the chicory root will help feed my microbiome. The dandelion root will help my liver do its work. Maybe this will help my immune system, too, as mushrooms are well-known immune modulators. As I dig into this afternoon's hot cup of creamy chaga (I mix it with powdered MCT coconut creamer and unsweetened almond milk), I look up other medicinal benefits of the brew. Apparently, it provides a 20-percent reduction in immune cell damage in IBD and healthy people. Bonus! I just thought it tasted good. If you like bitter, earthy tastes with a creamy texture, maybe try chaga for yourself.

SUMMARY

You could do all of these things, do a few together, or do them one at a time and rotate. Depends on the damage done. You might need longer treatment. Remember the rule of thumb: it takes one month for every year you've had an issue. You can't rush treatment. Additionally, with the gut, there can be repeat offenses even when you try your best. I promote variety as different rem-

---

130 Prucksunand, C., Indrasukhsri, B., Leethochawalit, M., & Hungspreugs, K. (2001). Phase II clinical trial on effect of the long turmeric (*Curcuma longa Linn*) on healing of peptic ulcer. *The Southeast Asian Journal of Tropical Medicine and Public Health*, 32(1), 208–215.

edies and foods help in different ways. Variety also helps you maintain your interest in following a lifelong gut-healing regimen.

As Stephen Covey says, "Fast is slow and slow is fast." If you rush the healing process, it actually might end up taking longer, thanks to setbacks and shortcomings. Take the protocol slow and steady, like the tortoise, and you will win. Take it fast, like the hare, and you will fall behind and maybe even give up. Don't give up. With some smart work and perseverance, you will end up much further ahead. Bowel-wise, mood-wise, spirit-wise. You'll be wiser. That's a good thing. After all, we are on a journey to learn things and become wise. That's what we're here to do.

Remember, this initial plan touches on how to clean up what has passed and prepare you for what is yet to come.

You might feel like there is an insurmountable mountain in front of you. Pause. Take a moment and realize how far you have come. You are already partway up! Take some time for yourself. Make a nice cup of herbal tea. Sit outside if you can. Breathe the fresh air and feel the sunshine.

Arrange for some professional guidance. But *you* must own the plan. Plan for success. Plan for failure. Failure happens. Athletes learn how to fall before they learn how to fly through the air.

Remember, there are many sub-layers to your health. When you peel things off like Band-Aids, it can hurt a little. In the next chapter, you'll learn how to prevent and recover from challenges.

CHALLENGES, HANG-UPS, AND HOLDBACKS

Here's what you'll learn in this chapter:

- Peel into your emotional layer
- Outsmart food cravings
- Food or mood—which comes first?
- Importance of blood sugar regulation
- Recognize and deal with emotional eating habits
- Have compassion for times of stress
- Moderation

"It's easy to conquer others; what's difficult is to conquer the self."

—BUDDHA

You can have all the plans in place, but until you put them into action, they are not going to serve you. You can't get healthy just by reading this. Boy, do I wish you could! It is going to take some effort on your part. That means changing some of your routines. Some find it easy to change them all at once. For most, it works better to focus on one area at a time and layer the changes. As with anything new, there are bound to be things that challenge you, things you have trouble incorporating. You may have difficulty letting go of old habits, even if they don't serve you anymore.

If you have a very messed-up microbiome and a leaky gut, your food sensitivity test may show that practically every food you eat is inflammatory. Eliminating most of your favourite foods is a shock to your system, and it is a challenge to find new appealing foods to substitute while your immune system calms down. Take it slow and be very patient with yourself. If you have struggled with an eating disorder in the past, restricting foods may be a trigger. Be careful!

One of the biggest challenges people face is their emotional relationship with food. Food is a social event. Food is a comfort. Food can also be an avoidance factor when you don't want to deal with your emotions. As with gambling, sex, shopping, and alcohol, you can get addicted to food.

FOOD CRAVINGS

NUTRIENT ABSORPTION

An imbalanced microbiome not only makes you fat but addicts you to unhealthy foods. If the body is not physically capable of absorbing the nutrients it needs, it craves what it cannot get. This can lead to nonsensical eating patterns.

The gut lining could be compromised by food sensitivities or inflammation from too many gram-negative bacteria, parasitic infections, stress overload, you name it. If the lining is not healthy, it cannot do its job well.

Food or mood—which comes first? It depends. We can sometimes legitimately get hungry. Your body sends plenty of messages to the brain. Then the brain interprets, but it doesn't always get it right.

THIRST

Sometimes we mistake hunger for thirst. We eat instead of drinking a tall glass of water. It is amazing how many people just drink coffee all day and never water. Coffee and regular tea don't hydrate the body. If your cells are all shrivelled up and the fluid around them is sticky because it doesn't have enough water, you are not going to feel so well. Dehydration can lead to low mood as your metabolism slows and lowers your energy. Low energy may trigger the signal that you need food when you really need water. Try drinking a large glass of water or having a cup of herbal tea and waiting five minutes before you decide if you are truly hungry.

On the other hand, you can drink too much water. The old adage of eight glasses of water a day isn't necessarily the golden rule. You will get water through herbal tea, soup broths, and some vegetables such as cucumber, squash, and celery. That counts. Your body is about 80 percent water and your stool 74 percent, so good, clean, filtered water is important. Water can be a source of toxins such as lead (from pipes) and hormones (runoff of pesticides, prescription medications flushed down the toilets), so be sure your source is as pure as possible. Drink from glass or stainless steel, not plastic!

EMOTIONAL HUNGER

Emotional hunger should not be confused with genuine craving. Your body is smart. Sometimes cravings serve as a means to satisfy deficiencies or imbalances. If you eat something you crave and then are satisfied with a small amount of the food, this is a genuine craving based on physical need. You may not crave the food again for a while. If you crave a food and can't stop eating it, it is likely an emotional craving, which food will have difficulty satisfying.

LEPTIN

Wheat, as we talked about before, can instill an opioid-like addiction to its gluteomorphins. To make matters worse, if you are sensitive to wheat, you may also have a leptin binding issue. That means wheat makes you eat constantly. I believe I have this. Not only does wheat cause blood sugar regulation issues, its proteins can actually bind to leptin and prevent it from reaching its receptor. Leptin is the signal that goes to the brain to say you have had enough to eat. If the signal doesn't get there, then you never feel satisfied. Leptin is also suppressed when there are high levels of cortisol. This might explain why some people overeat when they are stressed.

GHRELIN

Ghrelin is a hormone your stomach releases to stimulate appetite. You can remember this because *ghr*elin makes your stomach *gr*umble. An excess of ghrelin is released between meals to trigger hunger. Interesting that it is also released during sleep deprivation. Think of how hungry you get those nights staying up late to get work done. You eat, but really, you need sleep instead. Go to bed!

CAFFEINE

Caffeine and sugar are addictive substances. Wean off; it is easy to stay away. There are plenty of hot beverage alternatives. A cup of coffee can be a cup of stress. It causes spikes in adrenaline, which the body registers as stress. A little bit gets you going. Too much, and you wind up on a roller coaster. Up, down, need some more, can't sleep, drink coffee to wake up, have a second or third cup to really get things moving, can't sleep...Caffeine has a five-hour half-life. That means it takes five hours for half of it to power down. That's why the effects of one cup in the morning can last all day and why, if you have a cup in the afternoon, you will be awake at night. The same goes for tea, chocolate, energy drinks, anything with caffeine. You'd think we'd be smarter than this. You have the power to stop the crazy cycle.

Genetic components dictate why some people can handle more caffeine than others. Be honest about what works for you. There are plenty of antioxidants in tea and coffee. That's good. But when you are stressed, your body is busy detoxing from all the stress hormones, and adding caffeine to the mix adds to your problem. That's when you can rely more on blueberries, bilberries, or pomegranates for your antioxidant load.

CHOCOLATE

Chocolate can be a challenge for some. It's a caffeine hit, yes, but the proteins in chocolate and coffee can cross-react with gluten. Therefore, a gluten intolerance may lead to a coffee or chocolate intolerance. For those who can tolerate it, chocolate provides a good boost of nutrients, especially magnesium and a little iron. Two squares of dark chocolate a few days a week can boost your energy and mood; theobromine and phenylethalmine (PEA), an amphetamine-like stimulant, act as antidepressants.

IRON AND B12

Do you crave red meat? It is high in minerals and protein. If you're pregnant, your body needs a ton more iron to build blood for you and your baby.

Restless legs at night may be another sign of low iron. Meat also contains B12, which may help ease insomnia and depression. Over the past few weeks, I gave a weekly B12 shot to a patient to help with fatigue, and what do you know? After the first week, she started sleeping better at night and feeling less fatigued during the day!

PICA

Sometimes people crave the strangest things. Like dirt. Pica is the name of cravings for nonfood items, including the ingestion of earth (geophagy), raw starch (amylophagy), and ice (pagophagy). In addition to teaching you some new Scrabble words, these nonfood cravings are related to anemia, low hemoglobin and hematocrit concentration, and low zinc concentration.[131] Pica is suggestive of micronutrient deficiencies. If you have a compromised gut lining (leaky gut) for any length of time, you may deplete your body stores of essential minerals. Heal the gut and consider a high-quality bioabsorbable multimineral. A liquid one or a capsule might be nice so you don't have to do the extra work to break down the binding chemicals in a tablet.

SALT

Crave salt? Your adrenals are likely weak (blood pressure low) and need support. If you experience daily bouts of diarrhea (irritable bowel syndrome [IBS], irritable bowel disease [IBD], parasitic infection), be really careful to replenish your sodium. An electrolyte mix may be needed short term. Salt is essential for the nervous system. Fatigue, low mood, muscle aches, cramps, sleeplessness, and inability to concentrate are signs of low sodium.

Sodium gets a bad rap from the heart-health-conscious groups, but it depends on your tolerance (genes) and intake level. Diets higher in meat will naturally supply more sodium than plant-only diets. Highly processed foods, such as crackers, chips, cheese, breads, and deli meats, have a ton of salt. The goal is to eat more whole fresh foods, a lot of vegetables and some meat. When eating a home-cooked meal, you may use the salt shaker at the table to taste and not have an issue.

---

131 Miao, D., Young, S. L., & Golden, C. D. (2015). A meta-analysis of pica and micronutrient status. *American Journal of Human Biology*, 27(1), 84–93. https://doi.org/10.1002/ajhb.22598

"Sugar meltdown" is pretty plain to see in a young child. Give them some candy, a chocolate bar, ice cream, or cake, and watch what happens to their personality and behaviour in about thirty minutes. A well-behaved, polite child can turn into wild child.

Grown-ups are not much different. Take Catherine, for example. She's a 24-year-old nurse. She likes to go out and have a good time with her friends. This often involves drinking and junk food. She knows better, but it's one of her "vices." She came in and told me about the complete meltdown she'd had after a night out with the girls. She drank a number of canned vodka mixes and ate gummy bears and chocolate-covered almonds. The next day, it was more than a hangover. It was a complete SOS mood meltdown with uncontrollable crying, diarrhea, and feelings of very low self-worth. Two days later, her face broke out. She is still reeling from the event. Sugar meltdowns are real! Catherine is not alone in this experience. Maybe you feel the same way after a sugar binge. Even without the alcohol, sugar can make you feel so out of sorts you think you are beyond hope. You are not. There is lots of hope for you, especially if you realize what sugar does to you, and you stop eating it.

Sugar intake, microbiome imbalance, and cortisol (stress) spike inflammation and weaken the immune system. More inflammation spikes, more cortisol. Cortisol release gets you revved up. Long-term cortisol release increases insulin production, which leads to fat storage around the waist, giving you those unlovable love handles. If abused, the stimulus to manage insulin, and ultimately blood sugar, fails. This is called type 2 diabetes. It is mostly reversible with a gut reset protocol as described in this book.

Inflammation and chronic cortisol release can deplete the production of serotonin, GABA, and vitamins necessary to balance your mood. Evidently, anxiety and depression are not necessarily conditions unto themselves; they can be symptoms of an unhealthy gut.

If insulin puts sugar into storage, then what takes it out? Glucagon. Glucagon works opposite to insulin. It pulls energy out of cellular storage, increases blood sugar, and encourages fat burning. It is active between meals, when you are fasting, and when you are on a keto diet. Regular exercise and a balanced microbiome will help regulate glucagon.

Good microbes help make the serotonin you need. Foods that boost serotonin include butternuts, black walnuts, pecans, plantains, banana, avocado, pineapple, eggplant, and plums. Additionally, eat foods high in tryptophan (used to make serotonin) such as turkey and milk products away from other proteins to avoid competition for access to the brain. Foods high in B vitamins or magnesium such as meat, seafood, nuts, seeds, and dark leafy greens support the production of tryptophan and, ultimately, serotonin. Whole grains are a good source of B vitamins, too, although they are often hard on the gut, especially for those who are sensitive and whose gastrointestinal lining needs time and care to heal.

A craving for sweetness could be a need for protein. Protein slows the body's absorption of sugars and helps you feel full longer so you are more satisfied with your meal. If you crave sugar, eat some protein, such as a handful of almonds or a piece of chicken, and see how you feel five or ten minutes after.

Too much sugar and too much alcohol both lead to a fatty liver. Furthermore, sugar cravings often spike after you drink. When the muscle stores are full of energy, the liver packs it in; when the muscle stores are full of energy, the liver takes the overflow and starts to store it as fat. Additionally, the liver must work hard to detoxify alcohol. If it is busy doing that, it struggles to do its daily detox tasks. Red eyes, headaches, aggressive mood, anger, outbursts, and irritability can all be signs of poor blood glucose regulation in diabetics or those with a stressed liver. Alcohol temporarily relaxes, but in the long term, it can increase the risk of anxiety and depression. Detoxing it depletes B vitamins; this can contribute to depression and anxiety.

Alcohol can also be a substance of avoidance. When you take on more than you can emotionally digest, alcohol can numb the feelings. When you numb your emotions, you are not processing and releasing them. Emotions suppressed now will rear their heads later. It is also very difficult to heal the gut while drinking alcohol. Best to abstain while doing the gut reset.

THINGS TO HELP REDUCE CRAVINGS
TYROSINE

Lean pork, lean beef, chicken, and turkey are all sources of protein that include the amino acid tyrosine. Tyrosine boosts levels of two brain chemicals, dopamine and norepinephrine, which help keep you alert, focused, and satisfied.

CHOLINE

Choline helps reduce any craving. Why? It elevates brain dopamine levels.[132] More chicken skin, please! Everyone in our house fights over the crispy chicken skin. It tastes great, but who knew it was so good for us? Choline is used to build cell membrane structure (phospholipids), lipid transport (lipoproteins), and cleanse the liver.[133] It is also important for memory and reduces the risk of neural tube defects during pregnancy. Increased intake of choline can help reverse nonalcoholic fatty liver disease. Great sources of choline include egg yolks, chicken skin, beef, chickpeas, mung beans, and shiitake mushrooms.

GYMNEMMA

Cravings for sweetness are strong. It can be as addictive as cocaine.[134,135,136] An excess of sugar rewires the dopamine receptors in your brain. Outthinking your craving can be really tough. Cravings for sweets or alcohol could also be caused by a *Candida* overgrowth. *Candida* preferentially feeds itself by making you crave sugar.

A few drops of a tincture from *Gymnemma sylvestre*, an ancient Ayurvedic herb, can deter the taste buds from sweet temptations.

---

132 Renshaw, P. F., Daniels, S., Lundahl, L. H., Rogers, V., & Lukas, S. E. (1999). Short-term treatment with citicoline (CDP-choline) attenuates some measures of craving in cocaine-dependent subjects: A preliminary report. *Psychopharmacology*, 142(2), 132–138. https://doi.org/10.1007/s002130050871

133 Zeisel, S. H., & da Costa, K. A. (2009). Choline: An essential nutrient for public health. *Nutrition Reviews*, 67(11), 615–623. https://doi.org/10.1111/j.1753-4887.2009.00246.x

134 Rorabaugh, J. M., Stratford, J. M., & Zahniser, N. R. (2015). Differences in bingeing behavior and cocaine reward following intermittent access to sucrose, glucose or fructose solutions. *Neuroscience*, 301, 213–220. https://doi.org/10.1016/j.neuroscience.2015.06.015

135 Ahmed, S. H., Guillem, K., & Vandaele, Y. (2013). Sugar addiction: Pushing the drug-sugar analogy to the limit. *Current Opinion in Clinical Nutrition and Metabolic Care*, 16(4), 434–439. https://doi.org/10.1097/MCO.0b013e328361c8b8

136 Lenoir, M., Serre, F., Cantin, L., & Ahmed, S. H. (2007). Intense sweetness surpasses cocaine reward. *PloS One*, 2(8), e698. https://doi.org/10.1371/journal.pone.0000698

After taking a few drops a couple of times a day, or just when you crave sweets, you'll find your cravings have subsided. Even candy lovers enjoy sweet success with *Gymnemma*. Reputation from Ayurvedic medicine and more recent scientific research tells us that taken over longer periods, it can help lower blood sugar.[137] This likely is because when you take it, you no longer enjoy the taste of eating sweet things.

TREAT ISN'T ALWAYS EAT

It's not that you'll never be able to have a little sweetness. After being away from simple sugars or processed foods of any kind for three or four weeks, you will be much more sensitive to even tiny amounts of sweetness. With the change in the microbiome from the gut reset, you will no longer crave sweets the same and will get satisfaction from different kinds of treats. Treat does not always mean eat. There are other ways to show yourself love: a swim in the ocean, a new magazine, tea date with a friend, hike in a new park, a golf or squash game, massage, sound therapy, meditation, watching a funny movie, an art class, an afternoon of live theatre, or acupuncture can all be quite a treat! The ways in which you enjoy life shouldn't get in the way of enjoying life.

"Changing people's habits and ways of thinking is like writing instructions in the snow during a snowstorm. Every twenty minutes, the instructions must be rewritten, unless ownership is given along with instructions."

—JOHN C. MAXWELL

137 Tiwari, P., Mishra, B. N., & Sangwan, N. S. (2014). Phytochemical and pharmacological properties of *Gymnema sylvestre*: An important medicinal plant. *BioMed Research International, 2014*, 830285. https://doi.org/10.1155/2014/830285

EMOTIONAL EATING

Sometimes it's the mood, not the food, that comes first. Emotional eating is common. You might not even think you have an emotional tie to food. You do. Boredom and loneliness top the list for causes of emotional eating. We touched on this earlier, but let us expand more now.

If you are simply bored and eat in place of doing something interesting, focus instead on being creative. We all need purpose and passion. Pick a hobby. Cook, craft, volunteer, paint, colour. You don't have to be good at it. It's just a form of expression. As you engage in a creative process, you will be amazed how the time flies, and you won't even feel hungry. You might find it helpful to leave notes for yourself to remind you what to do before eating. Buy a pack of sticky notes and put them on the bag of cookies, the cupboard, the fridge. Put "Go for a walk," "Draw a picture," "Call a friend" or have a love list of things to do so you can start loving to do them. Then you won't be bored; you'll feel a sense of accomplishment and you'll learn the difference between feeling bored and being hungry.

For a long time, I would have to pause and say to myself, "Are you hungry or anxious?" Of course, I'd pick hungry. I like to eat! Feeling hungry is a good excuse to eat, right? It is, if you haven't eaten in a while and it is lunchtime. It's not, if you just ate a substantive meal, and now your brain says you are hungry. No go. I taught myself to pause for a minute and ask, "*Am I hungry or anxious?*" Then wait. Then ask, "*When did I last eat? Is it possible I am not hungry? Is it possible that I am anxious?*" Denial tries to lean into the hunger again. The next question I ask is, "*What just went through my mind? What thought came just before I said, 'I'm hungry'?"* It helps, by the way, to say *"I'm hungry"* out loud. Then you hear yourself. Your subconscious hears your conscious. It's harder to deny things this way.

At first, it is difficult to recognize the thought that comes before the feeling. A little like trying to catch a chipmunk. You see it, think you saw it, but *whoosh*, now it's vanished out of sight. Work at sneaking up on it, and you can feel its silky fur brush through your hands. Thoughts are like this. Work on coaxing thoughts. Slow them down a little. Tame them. Then you can catch them more easily. Find out what thought just went through your mind before you felt hungry. Ah. Okay. Could that thought have made you anxious? There we go. You're not hungry. You're anxious. Now, decide whether to take that thought and see why it made you anxious or just let it be. See if it goes away forever or pops back in again. Thoughts that pop in over and over need to be flushed out into the open and pulled apart. A chat with a friend, a psychotherapist, doctor, or a workbook such as *Mind over Mood* could help.

For anxiety that comes and goes, perhaps you need to reframe what's going on in your world. Reframing a situation gives you a renewed perspective. There will always be things that drive you NUTS. You had best learn how to deal with them. I learned this acronym when I studied with Chris Kresser. I think he got it from someone else. I can't remember who gets the ultimate credit. It's a keeper, though. Here it is: N for novel, U for unpredictable, T for threat (to the body or the ego), and S for a sense of loss. Here's how I interpret it.

Novel: If you encounter something that has never happened

before, how could you possibly know how to deal with it? It's new to you. So you have to be patient with yourself. Of course, you don't know how to deal with it. Naturally, you might ask a friend or a family member if they have ever dealt with something similar. Learn how they dealt with it. You might not choose to handle it in the same manner, but at least you won't feel alone, and you'll have some sense that others have been here before. You may also seek professional advice. Read a book on the new problem you have. Then make an educated decision on what is best for you.

Unpredictable: By definition, unpredictable things are those for which you're not prepared. You can learn from them so you won't be caught off guard by similar events in the future. Accidents and surprises are unpredictable by nature. Be patient with yourself when dealing with them. Do what you can to prepare for the future without pressuring yourself to prevent every accident or mishap—that's impossible.

Threat: When you feel under threat or on the defensive, try to understand why. What has made you feel threatened? Is it your ego rising? You will know it is when your guard goes up and you feel like attacking someone. You feel like you have been "wronged" or "put down" or simply feel like punching the other person in the face. It happens. We all have ego. It's not our best side. Recognize your feeling of anger, frustration, or lack of self-worth. You should never ignore these feelings, but you shouldn't put them in charge either. It's best at this point to simply check in with yourself. Ask, "Is there actually a threat here?" What advice would you give someone facing a similar situation? Sometimes a feeling of being threatened is justified. Sometimes there is good reason to feel you are not safe. If this is the case, you need to seek safety. Remove yourself from the situation, or get help to do so. From a new point of safety, evaluate the situation. Get help from family, friends, or professional organizations to rebuild your community of trust and well-being.

Sense of loss: This could be loss of a job, a home, a friend, a loved one, or even a routine. It is important to grieve the things you leave behind so you can be ready to accept what comes next.

If you follow the main principles of a healthy biorhythm, as discussed in the next chapter, you will find yourself more accepting to change.

Find calm within, and you can draw others into your sea of calm. This is a whole lot more productive than getting sucked into someone else's negative vortex. Be careful.

NAP TRAP

Stuck in the NAP trap? NAP stands for numb, avoid, or procrastinate.

An unmet emotional hunger can stem as far back as the first few years of life. Or it could have originated more recently. If you're deprived of love, hunger for this love is so powerful it drives you to elsewhere to quench it: food, sex, work, gambling, spending, or obsessive control over your environment. Human love is imperfect, so there is always room for abandonment and disappointment.

No one person is ever meant to completely fulfill you. You resonate your own happiness based on your own energies. You get your renewed sense of energy by feeling love *for* someone or something, not by feeling love *from* someone. It is nice when love is reciprocated. That doesn't always happen. It's not meant to. As hard as it is, sometimes it is time to move on. Just remember, you take yourself with you everywhere you go. If you drag unprocessed emotions around with you, you are no better than Linus with his stinky blanket. If this sounds like you, you might like to read *Wherever You Go, There You Are* by Jon Kabat-Zinn.

You want to numb your feelings, so you eat. You look for answers to your problems. You eat. Or drink. You want to relax. You have a glass of wine or a beer, or a big bowl of comfort food, or you dip into your secret stash. Give the power to the food, and it fails to solve anything. Then you feel even more let down. Sounds kind of silly, but it's true. The trouble is, the answer isn't in the bottom of the bag of cookies or chips. It's not even at the bottom of the ice-cream container.

The answer is within you.

Fear stops you from accessing your inner wisdom. Loneliness puts a roadblock in front of your heart.

Food can also be a pleasure-seeking expedition. It temporarily provides a physical distraction from the inner critic. But then, what happens? That inner critic beats you up for what you just ate. Not too nice now, is it?

This unmet emotional hunger needs to be recognized. Emotions need to be felt. They should neither be ignored nor placed in charge. How you feel is real to you, and it cannot be denied. Emotional pain is felt physically. The tightness in the heart. Ever felt pain in your heart as if an animal had reached in deep with its snarly claws and tore your beating heart right out of its cage? Like you want to cry, but you can't? You feel rejected and envision the stone-wall construction. One heavy painstaking rock at a time, you build around your heart to protect it from ever getting hurt again. Or you eat soft, cool ice cream to try and soothe the pain. Love lies deep in a broken heart. Let it surface. Give it time. It will be more precious than it was at the start.

Learn to love your emotions, to put love on them, to soothe them, as if you hold the small child inside of you with compassion and understanding. Allow the emotions to be.

Feel angry? Love that you recognize something is not working for you. Figure out a way you can act to change what you don't like into something that is better for everyone involved. Anger fuels motivation to act. That's its purpose. It took me a long time to understand and accept anger. People pleaser that I am, I didn't allow myself to feel angry. Instead, I became passive and aggressive. There was a time when I was afraid that if I got angry with someone, I might lose their love. Let me tell you, it works so much better to kindly tell the other person how you feel. Kindness is truth delivered with compassion and love. Anger can have love. But first, you have to feel your feelings and transform the angry energy to love energy.

Feeling tough feelings is hard work. It hurts. Since ours is a pleasure-seeking society, hurt is something we try to make go away. Or we try to run away from it. If we keep numbing the feeling, or avoiding it, or procrastinate dealing with it, it *never* resolves. You can try to make excuses about it, find ways to distract yourself, but it never ever goes away until you fully deal with it. If you stuff too much down for too long, it creates stress in your body. Stress tips your nervous system so that it shifts to a chronic state of fight or flight. That means less room to digest the food you eat, not to mention the chronic release of cortisol.

What about the helicopter parents who care for or control their children too much? Is it possible that parents who try to control their child's every move, set the stage for food rebellion? Yes. Food addictions are often a result of being held too tightly under "the law." Children who are not allowed to make guilt-free decisions rebel; food addictions and compulsive spending are often reactions that surface later in life.

LESSONS IN MODERATION

I just visited the West Coast. Along a lovely seaside town, there are a string of small craft breweries. Not just beer but kombucha and mead, too. Parents getting off the high-speed train from the day of work in the big city walk to the strip and meet up with local friends and family. In the back of the brewery is a yard with a chain-link fence and a thick coat of wood chips. Picnic tables overflow with people of all ages. It's not particularly warm out. My hands are cold and my cheeks are flush. The kids are running around playing tag. Colouring books, Barbie dolls, and homework are scattered on the tables. Parents standing, sitting. Some drink beer, some kombucha. Some wine or water. Kids have their canteens full of something brought from home. It's a real social event. Casual. Friendly. In this environment, drinking happens around the children, but it is not excessive. It is a beer or two, or a glass of wine. Or no alcohol, just a water or kombucha. Maybe a tray of fresh shucked oysters. Then, after an hour or two, home. Children raised in this environment will have a good chance of understanding the responsible and social side of drinking. They will understand that you don't have to drink to be social and that alcohol is not taboo. Moderation is key. A healthy message, permanently etched.

What if the message you received about food is not so healthy? What if it was used as your only reward? Or to keep you quiet? Some people actually carry extra weight around so it can act as a physical buffer. Do you eat to create a layer of physical protection? Instead of building that wall out of stones, do you build it out of chocolate cake? Tune in and ask yourself. Don't be harsh. You have to understand the five-year-old you and love it unconditionally. I say five, but it could be any age at which you had a traumatic experience. It is easy for us to freeze emotional development when we experience an overwhelming situation. This could be a move, a death, a divorce, abuse, or bullying. Anything you didn't have the maturity or skillset to process at the time. It's not your fault. It happened to you then. What is essential is to listen for what it may be for you, and recognize it so you can grow through those years you emotionally missed and catch up to who you are and who you'd like to be today. If eating to soothe isn't working so well for you anymore, time for new skills. If you need help with this, counsellors and psychotherapists are trained to guide you through the process. You don't need to know where to begin. Just show up and say you think you need some help. You can learn how to better regulate emotions and connect to your heart in chapter 9. Heart inspiration is key to intuitive intelligence and long-lasting energy. It is stronger than will power.

Connection with your heart can help you feel authentic and grounded. It lets you get messy in your feelings so you can let them go. Like when you dump the contents of your junk drawer out on the table. It has to be done before you can start to sort things out. I admit, I have not mastered this process. It's always easier to distract ourselves or to put our own issues aside to help someone else, or to process things logically, in the mind, without feeling them in the heart.

We are not perfect, but in our imperfection, we are perfectly who we are supposed to be. Right now. Who else are we going to be if we are not ourselves? Think of it this way: instead of expecting the party to be there for you so you can show up and be entertained, embrace what you have and bring it to the party. Get the difference?

"People who own their own lives

do not feel guilty when they make choices

about where they are going."

—CLOUD AND TOWNSEND[138]

You might feel a bit raw right now. Allow it. Accept it. Sit with it. There are times when we have to learn to be comfortable with the uncomfortable.

Go slow, though. Give your subconscious time to process what's coming up. You are peeling back the layers. We need to do this

---

138 Cloud, H., & Townsend, J. S. (1992). *Boundaries: When to say yes, when to say no to take control of your life.* Zondervan.

in stages. While that's cooking on the back burner, engage in something creative: garden, listen to some music, walk in nature, colour, or breathe and meditate.

When you are ready, come on back. We'll have a look at how sleep and biorhythms impact your gut in the next chapter. Then I'll loop back to feelings with you.

RHYTHM AND BLUES

Here's what you'll learn in this chapter:

- Why can't I sleep? How gut reactions affect your ability to fall and stay asleep.
- What happens in the gut while we sleep?
- Circadian rhythms—400x more melatonin is made in the gut than the brain. What's that about?
- Tips for better sleep
- Travel, jet lag, and irregular bowels—what to do about it
- Food volume and timing affect the gut
- Benefits of digestive rest, often helpful on its own, for a digestive reset when an intestinal flare occurs
- Tips for fasting—how long, what's safe, who's safe?

"Sleepiness happens when the conscious mind has absorbed as much as it can and needs time to digest the material."

—PENNEY PEIRCE

I love how it feels to lie on the salty seawater. Thanks to the increased buoyancy, it is possible to float around for hours. The rhythm of the waves could rock me to sleep. We are all made of energy, and ultimately, energy is a wave. Ocean wave, sound wave, light wave, microwave, electromagnetic wave. Every cell in your body oscillates at a certain wavelength.

There are natural rhythms or waves that are daily, tidal, weekly, seasonal, and annual. It is what our great creator manages at a universal level. The earth rotates on its axis; the moon rotates around the earth. The earth, moon, and all the planets rotate around the sun. The rotations bring us night and day. Monthly rhythms come with the moon's pull. Tides rise and fall in the ocean and the seas. Seasons change from spring to summer to fall to winter. All these rhythms churn us through time.

We have brain waves. The heart's beat can be measured in waves. The gut moves food down its channel in peristaltic waves (smooth muscles contract and release to propel food through the intestinal tract). External cues can adjust these natural and automatic bio-rhythms to the local environment. Another name for an external cue is "zeitgeber" (German for time giver). Zeitgebers include light, temperature, magnetic pull, food, and social activities.[139]

CIRCADIAN RHYTHM

Circadian rhythm is any biological wave that displays a pattern or repeated processes around a twenty-four-hour clock. Circadian

---

139 Rouleau, N., & Dotta, B. T. (2014). Electromagnetic fields as structure-function zeitgebers in biological systems: Environmental orchestrations of morphogenesis and consciousness. *Frontiers in Integrative Neuroscience*, 8, 84. https://doi.org/10.3389/fnint.2014.00084

comes from the Latin *circa*, which means around, or approximately, a certain time of day. Abnormal sleep-wake cycles and disruption of zeitgebers aggravate the circadian rhythm and make intestinal cells more vulnerable to injury. This also rings true for cellular waves. Waves we use for cell phones and internet Wi-Fi can have an impact on the waves we have in our human cells. This electromagnetic smog disrupts our sleep, making our cells more vulnerable to injury and disease. We already know sleep disruption can predict irritable bowel syndrome (IBS); 30 percent of those who worked a twenty-four-hour on-call shift in the past six months experience irregular bowel function (IBS) or indigestion, and 5 percent of the time, both.[140] Chronic circadian rhythm disruption, regardless of shift work, electromagnetic smog, blue light, or other zeitgeber zappers, is linked to gastrointestinal diseases such as IBS and colorectal cancer.

Traditional Chinese medicine beautifully teaches the endogenous (body-based or "home-made") clocks. It considers the twenty-four-hour clock of daily rhythms, five seasons of change, and a lifetime of chronological maturation.

Twenty-four-hour clocks are typically referred to as diurnal rhythms. We know these rhythms innately, just like the birds somehow know when it is time to fly south for winter. They are tuned into external cues such as light, temperature, and purification cycles. The human intestinal circadian rhythm influences gut movement, nutrient absorption, metabolism, and cell regeneration.

---

140 Lim, S. K., Yoo, S. J., Koo, D. L., Park, C. A., Ryu, H. J., Jung, Y. J., Jeong, J. B., Kim, B. G., Lee, K. L., & Koh, S. J. (2017). Stress and sleep quality in doctors working on-call shifts are associated with functional gastrointestinal disorders. *World Journal of Gastroenterology*, 23(18), 3330–3337. https://doi.org/10.3748/wjg.v23.i18.3330

Did you know that cells in the body regenerate every ten years? After ten years, you have an entirely new set of cells. A new you! For the gut, turnover is much faster—typically three days for most. The cyclical mechanisms or circadian rhythms affect all living things. That includes the microbes in our microbiome. They, too, have circadian rhythms of their own that will ultimately affect our human sleep-wake cycle, hormone release, and metabolism. These rhythms intersect and reflect one another, like the waves from two stones dropped in water. Watch the ripples meet each other at multiple points.

The twenty-four-hour daily rhythms describe how body organs are most active at different times of the day or night. If there is balance in the body, the circadian cycles dance to a harmonious beat that serves the body well. When timing gets off, organ function becomes imbalanced. For example, your deepest sleep should be at 2:00 a.m., lowest body temperature at 4:30 a.m., and a sharp rise in blood pressure and cortisol between 6:00 a.m. and 7:00 a.m. As the cortisol spikes, the melatonin drops. You are awake. The switch triggers the bowels to move. The highest testosterone release is at 9:00 a.m. The mental peak of alertness is at 10:00 a.m. The best coordination is at 1:30 p.m. Early afternoon brings a modest release of cortisol, which will see you through the rest of the day. The fastest reaction time is at 3:30 p.m., the greatest cardiovascular and muscle strength at 5:00 p.m. Highest blood pressure is at 6:30 p.m., and the highest body temperature is at 7:00 p.m. Melatonin secretion starts at 9:00 p.m., and bowel movements are suppressed by 10:30 p.m. If you are waking in the night between the hours of 1:00 a.m. and 3:00 a.m., I am going to bet you have a busy mind planning, making lists, and checking them twice. Unless you are Santa Claus, this list checking is not what you need to be doing in the middle of the night. The liver is overactive and needs to be calmed. Remove the obstacles to health, and rhythm will appear on its own.

Seasonal change brings focus to organ function. In winter, the kidneys, adrenals, and the urinary bladder need the most support. Springtime is the season for renewal, regeneration, detoxification—a perfect time to focus on support of the liver and gallbladder. Think of all the spring cleanup you do around your yard or in the city streets. Your body is no different. Winter is cold and stagnant, and once it ends, you and your house are in need of some fresh air and a good spring cleaning.

As spring matures, it lightens up into a warm, sunny summer. Now the heart, small intestine, pericardium (lining of the heart), and triple burner (digestive processes) are at their height of action. Summer is a prime time to heal the small intestine, which is naturally at the centre stage and most receptive during the warmer months. For the large intestine, the best time is in the fall, but first, there is an in-between season. As the height of summer wanes and the days begin to shorten, there is a touchdown to Earth. Spleen, pancreas, and stomach will awaken to have their needs met, and it is a time when the bounty and sweetness of ripened fruit is most welcome.

As the touchdown to Earth lifts onto the rails of fall, it is prime time to begin the support for the large intestine where more than 70 percent of the immune system resides. This transition time is when many people get a cold or flu. As the seasons change, the immune system needs support.

The tidal change of the monthly lunar or moon cycle brings ovulation at full moon and menstruation at new moon.

Without getting into a full-blown lesson on Chinese medicine, I hope you can appreciate that the ancients of over 2,000 years ago respected the natural biological clocks and had effective ways to bring balance to a body in a state of dis-ease. Modern science can attest to the biological rhythms. Research show humans do so much better going to bed before midnight and rising to have clear and focused minds early in the morning.

WHY CAN'T I SLEEP?

Sleep disruption can be temporary or long-standing. I always want to know how my patients are sleeping. What time to bed, what time to rise, how many times up in the night? How long to get to sleep at bedtime or after waking up in the night? Do you wake rested? What disturbs you or keeps you awake? How much caffeine (coffee, tea, chocolate, energy drinks) are you consuming? Do you have food sensitivities? Indigestion? Pain? Pets? A partner? What about room temperature, noise, light disturbances? Anxiety? Breathing issues? Sleep apnea? Snoring? Midnight snack?

Sleep supports the cognitive layer of your onion. When you sleep, your mind organizes events from the day and unprocessed emotions. If you are not sleeping, not much else is happening. You need sleep. Your body needs the day, and it needs the night, too. It is not an option, and it is not inactive. Many physical restorative functions are done on the body's night shift. If you don't sleep, your cognitive function declines.

Some studies find sleep deprivation can be as dangerous as driving drunk.[141]

An imbalanced microbiome can impair sleep. The microbiome bacteria normally make small quantities of toxins called lipopoly-saccharides and cellular chemicals called cytokines that induce your dream state (REM) sleep. An imbalanced microbiome can promote larger quantities of these toxins and chemical messengers, which will disrupt sleep, not to mention that the excess toxins can lead to inflammation and pain in the head, muscles, or joints. Pain keeps you up at night.

Cortisol, in its healthy biorhythm, interacts with the microbiome to induce a release of cellular biochemicals, which appear to help the body shift from early (non-REM) sleep to late sleep (REM/dream). During REM (rapid eye movement) sleep, we dream the deepest. Dream deprivation results in catastrophic breakdown of the human psyche. Dreams and sleep are keepers of our sanity.

"To sleep, perchance to dream: ay, there's the rub..."

—WILLIAM SHAKESPEARE, *HAMLET*

Circadian rhythm is linked to rises and falls of cortisol. In a natural rhythm, as the sun and cortisol goes down, the moon and melatonin rise. High cortisol messes with the microbiome. Low cortisol messes with the microbiome. You need cortisol to rise and fall on schedule to coordinate the proper biorhythms. A lovely, balanced wave.

---

141 Williamson, A. M., & Feyer, A. M. (2000). Moderate sleep deprivation produces impairments in cognitive and motor performance equivalent to legally prescribed levels of alcohol intoxication. *Occupational and Environmental Medicine*, 57(10), 649–655. https://doi.org/10.1136/oem.57.10.649

Gut rhythm is affected by stress (environmentally stimulated cortisol release), whether it be from infection and disease, irregular eating patterns, food composition, food sensitivities, antibiotics, alcohol, shift work, travel, jet lag, or sleep interruption. All of these contribute to intestinal hyperpermeability (leaky gut).

The basic way to tell if your cortisol is at a healthy level and in sync is to record when you eat, sleep, and go to the bathroom. Do you feel rested in the morning and have energy all day? Do you dream? This will tell you if your natural rise and fall of cortisol is balanced. If you have issues getting to sleep or staying asleep, don't feel rested in the morning, have poor functioning all day, and really dip in energy mid-afternoon, your cortisol levels may be out of whack. Chronic cortisol release can leave you feeling tired and wired. You want to sleep. You need to sleep. You can't sleep.

The scientific way to measure your cortisol and melatonin levels is to do a dried urine analysis and salivary test. The dried urine test is collected over twenty-four hours and measures all the breakdown products related to cortisol. The salivary test is done first thing in the morning and reveals cellular cortisol levels at their highest peak. Together, these results can shed light on your biorhythms. Things that can flatline your cortisol are very similar to those that flatline your microbiome. Stress, prescription drugs such as painkillers and corticosteroids, and poor thyroid function can all disrupt your body's natural routine. If you find your rhythms are off, the best way to start a reset is to take care of the gut, get lots of rest, and establish a daily routine of sleep, gentle exercise, and whole foods. Like a child's body, an adult body still needs the simple comforts of a daily routine. When life throws a curveball, get these things in check so your body can follow, or at least not fight, the example you set.

A problem with sleep sometimes comes for women in perimenopause. As the ovaries cease their ovulation duties, it takes a while for the body to catch up to the change. Surges and drops in hormones cause the telltale symptom of hot flushes, as well as new issues with constipation and poor sleep. That's because changes in estrogen affect the microbiome. I am not sure if scientists know exactly how lower levels of estrogen disrupt sleep. But studies do show estrogen therapy can help with sleep. Even homeopathic doses have worked for my patients.

WHAT HAPPENS IN THE GUT WHILE WE SLEEP?

Each gut microbe has its own circadian rhythm that tells it where to go in the gut and when. Different microbes might travel to different locations at different times. A bit like the birds in migration using their zeitgeber cues. They do this with very specific purpose. The timing provides windows of opportunity during which different microbes are more active. Depending on which microbes make which short-chain fatty acids at which time will determine which genes turn on and off. The genes then activate biochemical pathways both in the gut and throughout the entire body.

Thus, through these cyclical mechanisms, the biological clocks of the gut microbiome intimately intertwine with your own circadian rhythm. This regulates your sleep-wake cycles, hormone release, and metabolism. If the gut is out of order, so are you!

To keep a body running on schedule, all organs need to be synchronized with each other. Zeitgeber cues such as light, temperature, and food intake are strong signals. Clock feedback loops send messages to and from the brain. This master clock is called the suprachiasmatic nucleus. Circadian rhythm disruption is linked to many chronic diseases, including metabolic syndrome, obesity, cardiovascular disease, intestinal dysbiosis (IBS), inflammatory bowel disease (IBD), neurodegenerative diseases, and cancer.

Did you know you have 400x more melatonin in the gut than in the brain? It's true. Most think of the pineal gland's melatonin (in the brain), but that's only a tiny part of the picture. Melatonin is made in cells that line the stomach and extend down to the colon. The release is not light dependent. It may have something to do with gut microbe gene stimulation, as described above. Gut melatonin helps regulate digestion and food intake. There are also significant amounts of melatonin in bile, which is made by the liver and stored in the gallbladder.[142]

Melatonin can reach all cells in the body within minutes. It is very helpful not only in the circadian rhythm but also in free radical scavenging (think tumour reduction), protection of the gut lining and mucosa, and healing gastrointestinal lesions such as stomatitis, esophagitis, gastritis, peptic ulcer, and colitis. It improves immune function and triggers smooth muscles in the gastrointestinal tract. Melatonin helps rejuvenate gut cells. This is critical because, as you now know, they refresh every three to five days. Maybe that's why there is so much more melatonin in the gut than in the brain.

---

142 Reiter, R. J., Tan, D. X., Manchester, L. C., Gitto, E., & Fuentes-Broto, L. (2010). Gastrointestinal tract and melatonin: Reducing pathophysiology. *Gastroenterologia Polska, 17*(3), 213–218.

Brain melatonin is a bit different from gut melatonin. The brain melatonin is sensitive to light, especially blue light. Brain melatonin is released in the evening, when it starts to get darker outside and your cortisol, like the sun, dips down. You need this dip to get to sleep, and you need sleep to help regulate your entire circadian rhythm. So, ultimately, the brain melatonin will affect your gut melatonin's ability to work. If you see any blue light at all, it will prevent the melatonin from being released from the pineal gland. Melatonin is what makes you sleepy. This is the reason to start avoiding backlit screens at least an hour before bed and to remove cell phones from the bedroom. Also, cover up with electrical tape any blue light sensors on anything electric in the bedroom. Better yet, remove the electric interferences from the bedroom altogether.

Poor sleep is linked to reduction in melatonin. Melatonin plays a crucial role in regulating body temperature, sleep-wake cycle, female reproductive hormones, and cardiovascular function. Low melatonin is linked to anxiety, stress, depression, seasonal affective disorder, sleep disorders, immune disorder, cardiovascular disease, and cancer. High melatonin (without supplementation) is linked to inflammation in the brain.

When was the last time you stayed up late and then got sick? Sleep is critical to your immune defence. Different rates or times of day for cell rejuvenation may affect your ability to fight off infection. The bad guys—that is, the bacteria, viruses, fungi, and parasites— have picked up on this flaw in our immune system. In addition to factors of travel and sleep-wake cycle changes that mess with the gut rhythms and ultimately the immune function, the bad guys know that if they mess with the gut microbe clocks, they can get by the sentry guards of the immune system, get into the body, and start replication. This is how they spread infection.

Was staying up so late worth it? Next time, try going to bed at your regular hour and getting up with a fresh start in the morning. You will likely be more productive and healthier in the long run. That's how I got through life when I commuted daily for over an hour into the big city. To bed at nine and up at five. Every day. No exceptions. My mind was okay with it, too. The short-term memory worked hard at storage in my sleep and was fresh in the morning to double-check anything that didn't quite gel. I'd work out first thing in the morning, then eat breakfast and start my day. Going to bed, waking up, eating, and exercising at the same times every day helps your body keep a natural and healthy circadian rhythm. Get a hold of the day before it gets a hold of you! Our bodies LOVE routine. It is too bad we often view routine as boring! We need the proper rise and fall of cortisol to happen on schedule so the other biorhythms of the body coordinate.

If you do all this, you will be more focused and keep your biorhythms in check so you can concentrate and manage all the other things life throws at you. If you know you'll go to the bathroom about the same time every morning, doesn't that just make your day a tiny bit easier? It's amazing what the little things can do for you.

"Sleep is better than medicine."

—ENGLISH PROVERB

JOAN'S STORY

Joan looks like she is 52 when she walks into my office. She's 42. Her hair is greying, she has dark circles under her eyes, and her skin is dry and wrinkled. Her energy is low, and she wants help with sleep. She is on a leave from work as a business analyst because she could hardly function. Sleep is difficult and has been for months. At best, she gets two hours a night. She is so tired, but she cannot sleep. Averse to sleeping pills, she wants to see if there is a more natural solution. She's tried melatonin, sleepy time tea, herbal combinations, magnesium, no caffeine, staying in bed, getting up from bed. You name it, she'd tried it. Nothing worked. We decide to try the reverse sleep routine. She'd like to get up at seven o'clock and feel refreshed. In the past, she'd normally sleep seven hours solid. We count backwards from 7:00 a.m. for seven hours. That's midnight. The end goal is for her to be in bed before midnight. But we can't start there because that already is not working. We start with the number of hours she is currently sleeping soundly: two. To start, she stays up, out of bed until five o'clock, then goes to bed and sets the alarm for seven. The next night, she stays up until four. So long as she sleeps through the time she is in bed, she is allowed to increase the time in bed by thirty to sixty minutes. If she has issues sleeping, then she can back up to a shorter time for some nights until she sleeps through again. Joan does this until she is able to sleep seven hours straight without disturbance. Getting up once to go pee is allowed, so long as she is able to resume sleep within ten minutes. In Joan's case, we use external cues and sleep hygiene habits to reestablish her natural rhythms. It takes time, but it works.

In the appendix, there are some basic sleep hygiene habits. Pick three things you could implement over the next week. See what difference they make. Get those under your wing, and if you still need help with sleep, see what else you might be able to incorporate.

Sleep aids are not meant to be taken long term. The ones that are a type of antihistamine will make it difficult to lose weight. Some of the prescription ones are habit-forming and leave you groggy. Herbal passionflower, valerian, hops, skullcap, and catnip all can be helpful to calm the nervous system. If you choose to take these in a tea, do so two hours before bed. That way, you won't be up to the bathroom because of it. Some people are stimulated instead of calmed with valerian, so watch for that. You may also find these plant medicines in tincture or homeopathic form. Magnesium can be a real help, too. Ask your practitioner for some direction and see what suits your body best. So much healing happens in your sleep. It is important to establish a good night's sleep as part of your gut healing protocol.

MEAL TIMING

Ever noticed if you eat too late at night, it is difficult to get to sleep? A snack can be helpful, but a full-fledged meal doesn't sit so well once you lie down. There are natural rhythms to digestion. Your body has them. Your gut microbes have them. Everyone is operating on a cadence affected by zeitgebers. Your greatest wish is that they harmoniously ride the waves together. Imagine yourself like a surfer on the ocean. In order to stay afloat, your body has to move up and down and adjust to the waves.

FASTING

Time-restricted eating, such as most do for eight to twelve hours every night, can restore healthy cycling of the gut microbiota. If that doesn't work, fasting for an extended period can normalize out-of-sync gut microbe rhythms.[143] It can even reverse some negative effects associated with circadian disruption, such as insulin resistance.[144] This is crucial to control blood sugar and inflammatory factors. There is no one right way to fast. In his book *A Complete Guide to Fasting*, Jason Fung, MD, explains that barring the intake of food will eventually force the body to go to the fat stores to access that for energy. Insulin gets a break as it is not needed to counter the bolus of sugars coming from the digestive tract. Thus, fasting has been known to reverse type 2 diabetes.

Historically, fasting began as a natural expression of grief. Scripture describes fasting as "afflicting" one's soul or body (Isaiah 58:3-5). Many people of faith use periods of fasting to provide space for stronger spiritual connection. If you are interested in the history of fasting and types of spiritual fasting, Elmer Towns has a lovely read called *Fasting for Spiritual Breakthrough*. Here, again, you can see the link between the health of the gut, digestion, and greater aspects of being. I sometimes imagine the realms inside the gut like a spiritual fighting ground; it reminds me of Ephesians 6:12: "For we are not fighting against flesh-and-blood enemies, but against evil rulers and authorities of the unseen world, against might powers in this dark world, and against evil spirits in the heavenly places."

---

143 Manoogian, E., & Panda, S. (2017). Circadian rhythms, time-restricted feeding, and healthy aging. *Ageing Research Reviews, 39*, 59-67. https://doi.org/10.1016/j.arr.2016.12.006

144 Kaczmarek, J. L., Thompson, S. V., & Holscher, H. D. (2017). Complex interactions of circadian rhythms, eating behaviors, and the gastrointestinal microbiota and their potential impact on health. *Nutrition Reviews, 75*(9), 673-682. https://doi.org/10.1093/nutrit/nux036

"Starve a fever." Rest, fever, and fasting are part of the secret recipe to fight infection. Where does most of the war rage? At least 70 percent in the gut. You learned this. If the gut is busy digesting food, it struggles to focus on warding off infection. Our bodies are designed to heal themselves. Fasting helps unclog and free up the lymphatic system, which is where we find the other 30 percent of our immune defence.

Regardless, fasting can be a time to break away from feeding the physical body to connect and fill the void with the Spirit. We fast while we sleep. We dream. Through dreams, we connect with Spirit. If we are not digesting things of this world—emotions, food, or the energies of those around us—we have the full opportunity to digest the word and world of the Spirit. The state of fasting is a state of digestive rest. It is a state for spiritual connection.

"When we dream, we are in our natural state, which is spirit."

—DR. MARINA QUATTROCCHI

If I tell myself I am going to take a little digestive break, I am totally calm and ready for it. While the body digests food, it has to work pretty hard at producing all the enzymes, making the muscles work to chew, swallow, churn the stomach, mobilize the gastrointestinal tract, make nutrients, absorb nutrients, and produce hormones. It's like an assembly plant. If your assembly plant runs 24/7, eventually, it is going to need a break.

Naturally, one should not fast if pregnant or breastfeeding, nor if they have little fat to sustain themselves. Diabetics need to monitor their blood sugar and be medically supervised to ensure prescribed drug dosage is adjusted as their body's insulin regulation responds to the fasting.

Most important is to make sure you are fit to fast and drink plenty of water and herbal teas. No sweeteners, sugar, or fruit juices. Start your day with only your tea or coffee, if you drink one. No sugar or milk. You can try MCT (medium-chain triglyceride)—aka dried coconut milk—creamer. See what works well for you. It is safe to exercise and do anything you would normally do, so long as you feel okay. You can work through hunger pangs. Those will pass. If you feel woozy, nauseous, or unwell, eat.

Most start with intermittent fasting. This is where you stop eating after supper, and you don't eat until maybe ten or eleven o'clock the next day. If you get hungry, try to pace it out. This is not about starving yourself. It is not about deprivation. It is about digestive rest. If you do well starting to eat an hour after your regular breakfast time, then maybe the next day, you try going an hour longer. You can fast like this as many days of the week as makes sense for you, for as long as it continues to work.

GEORGE'S STORY

George, 49, comes to see me for weight issues and sleep. His wife complains he snores at night, and she is now sleeping in the other room. George misses having her at his side. Prone to anxiety, he likes to be able to reach over and know she is there through the night. Sometimes he wakes with a start and has troubles settling back to sleep. Since he was 35, George has gained 25 pounds. He has borderline blood sugar, and his blood pressure is creeping up. His medical doctor warned him the next step is medication. George wants to avoid this. We did his initial intake, diet diary, and body scan. George tries to stay away from the breads and pasta. He does his best to eat vegetables at lunch and dinner. I encourage George to get a sleep study done to rule out sleep apnea. It comes back borderline. If he loses some weight, he will decrease the excess fat around his neck and have less obstructing his breath while he sleeps. George is a good candidate for intermittent fasting. With it, he may have a chance to reverse his trend toward diabetes and heart disease.

George starts with delaying breakfast by one hour. Instead of eating at eight, he now eats at nine. He does this for a couple of weeks. He also takes note of his eating patterns at night. We go through the difference between physical and emotional food cravings. We work on HeartMath® breathing techniques. We will talk about HeartMath® more in chapter 10, but allow me to introduce it now. The HeartMath® company has studied the science of the heart since the early 1990s. They recognize that heart rate variability (HRV), or each beat-to-beat variation of the heart, is tied to a particular emotion. By training your heart through breath and mind focus techniques, you balance your nervous system, redirect emotions, lower blood pressure, boost immune response, enhance hormone balance, and better manage stress. You can track HRV with a device that hooks up to your ear and shows progress on a computer program. By seeing his results, George can tell when he makes a positive shift and, more importantly, learn how the shift feels in his body. He practices HeartMath® techniques for at least five to fifteen minutes a day, until the more balanced state becomes his new normal. He now goes to bed at ten and rises by seven.

After two weeks, George is doing well. He is not feeling deprived in the morning and is ready to extend his fasts. He decides to stop eating by eight at night and gradually extend his hours until breakfast in the morning. Over the course of three weeks, George is able to wait to eat until ten and sometimes even eleven. He loses 5 pounds.

George decides to replace his eleven-year-old mattress and freshen up his pillows. He buys a side sleeper to help keep him from rolling onto his back. In the evening, after dinner he goes for a walk for about twenty minutes. This is in addition to his weight and cardio workout in the morning. After his walk, he goes out into his shop to do some woodworking. The hobby helps keep his mind occupied and away from the kitchen. It also helps to think about the designs and creations when he wakes up anxious in the night.

Two months into the mission, George has lost 13 pounds. He now does his intermittent fasting five days a week. He is ready to try one or two days of longer fasting. He plans to keep his eating window to six hours. He chooses noon to six. At first, it is challenging. The first day, at eleven, he has to eat because he feels lightheaded and faint. He eats a handful of mixed salted nuts and drinks a big glass of water. It helps. Then he eats lunch at noon and has an apple in the afternoon and a good stir-fry vegetable with chicken and sweet potato for supper. A few days later, he tries the eighteen-hour fast again. It helps to call it an eating window. Soon, he gets the hang of it and does it for two or three days a week. At month five, he has lost a total of 18 pounds. At the six-month mark, George has his blood work repeated. His blood sugars are now in the normal range and his blood pressure has dropped as well. He is not waking anxious in the night so often anymore. His wife tries a few nights sleeping back with him and finds George's snoring has pretty well subsided.

George uses fasting to stimulate some weight loss and reset his gut microbiome and insulin levels. He didn't change a whole lot in his diet, but he did reduce his gluten intake and increased his vegetable intakes. He established daily routines for exercise and sleep. Until he achieves the results he seeks, he has two days a week of six-hour eating windows, three days of eight-hour eating windows, and two days of twelve-hour eating windows. This routine works for George. If he finds he loses too much weight, he can go back to eight-hour eating windows daily. If his weight or blood sugars rise again, he can reinstate the fasting regime as he sees fit. For George, this solution is a whole lot better than medications for life.

Are you confidently riding on the top of all those waves that regulate you and your microbiome's biological rhythms? Flow with it. You peeled the physical layer and removed obstacles to health. You touched the border where physical meets emotional with food or mood. With better sleep and routines, you strengthen the cognitive layer of health; with a healthy biorhythm, you will experience clearer thinking.

Take a moment to allow this wave of energy to propel you on a bike ride, a swim, a dance, or some time playing with the dog.

When you are ready to dig a little deeper, come back, and we'll peel into the layer of your inner onion. Warning: it could make you cry.

FLIGHT, FIGHT, FRIGHT, OR FREEZE

Here's what you'll learn in this chapter:

- Peel into the spiritual layer of the gut
- How fear and stress impact gut health
- The gut as a sensory organ
- The gut as your primary immune defence

Flight, fight, fright, or freeze, forgive...

What's your giant? Your fear? We all have them. New ones every day.

Why are these all F-words?! I'm not sure. How about faith? That's the strongest F-word ever. With it, you can conquer your fear. I'm talking faith as in the belief in an all-powerful creator. Why we have to think it is either big bang or Adam and Eve, I'm not sure.

Either way, it is a mystery, and maybe those are just two different ways of telling the same story.

First, your fear must be articulated. Stephen King, author of many very scary books, once said, "If a fear cannot be articulated, it can't be conquered."

Peel the onion.

We covered the physical-meets-emotional layer in the chapter on challenges to change. We know now how sleep and a healthy gut contribute to our memory and cognitive function. Dig a little deeper, and you will see how the health of the gut is tied to how we face our fears. Fear is film that builds between the emotional and spiritual layer.

FEAR AND STRESS

Fear is how we perceive a threatening situation. You have fear? You have stress in your body. To overcome fear, face it with an action plan. Face it with courage.

Take David and Goliath, for example. So many artists depict David as a meek shepherd boy, a young, prepubescent and with a feminine stature. They show him with his foot resting on the decapitated head of the giant Goliath. Victory after the slay. They tell nothing of what it took to slay that giant. It's just a given that David did it. How could this young, meek boy do this? I gather one could argue he did so with the strength and power of God. Sure. I get that. But consider Michelangelo's depiction of David. Contrary to convention, he depicted David in the image of how he imagined God, a perfectly crafted male pillar of muscles and strength. Most of all, what you see in the eyes and body language of David shows the courage it takes to face any fear. You show courage when you decide to face your fear and take the first step forward. It's not that you behead the giant. It's that you decide you have the strength within you to face the fear. That's what matters.

Courage modulates cortisol.

Cortisol is your stress hormone. Fear and stress mount a cortisol reaction. Long-term fear keeps the cortisol pumping through your body like water through a firehose fighting a five-alarm fire. You cannot continuously fight a five-alarm fire and not get burned.

A healthy development of gut microbiota is required for the normal development of the hypothalamic-pituitary-adrenal (HPA) axis. Gut microbes contribute to the quality of sleep and stress reactions; they influence hypothalamic roles in memory, mood, and cognition.

The pituitary is the master gland of your endocrine (hormone) system. Disruption in gut balance affects your hormone function. When constant or repeated stress stimulates the HPA axis, the adrenal glands release large amounts of cortisol. After prolonged periods of cortisol release, sometimes the adrenals get depleted and the body is unable to properly respond to stress. If the HPA axis is out of order, chances are, your gut and blood sugar regulation are out of order, too.

A few summers ago, my adrenals crashed. I did the DUTCH hormone test (dutchtest.com) and my cortisol was flatlined. My blood sugar regulation was really out of order. Magnesium and adrenal support were super helpful, but initially, I was up in the night to eat because I couldn't draw upon any stores I had. Cortisol is used to take sugar out of stores and into the bloodstream. Without it, you will need to be on a slow trickle of food to provide energy just in time. Nighttime hypoglycemia (low blood sugar) includes nightmares, crying in sleep, excessive sweating, or feeling tired, irritated, or confused upon waking.

Our innate survival mechanisms are geared to help us acquire food. Our cat lets the whole house know if she is running low on food. She is a real bowl-half-empty kind of girl. We call it the five-star kitty alarm. With such strong food sensitivities, I know how she feels; sometimes I have food security issues, too.

This sense of food insecurity mounts with travel. Emergency snacks, meal planning...there is an entire food strategy. I used to be really bad with this when my insulin regulation was a bit of a disaster. For years, I didn't even know what was going on. I'd be in business meetings all gung-ho, then tank halfway through them. Like a deflated balloon. Not so cool. Or I'd go out shopping and struggle to stand and walk around for any length of time without having something to eat. I started with butterscotch candies. Then I went healthier, and a bag of almonds was always with me. I'd take a three-day supply of food with me on a five-hour flight. After working through a strategy very much like what I talk about in this book, I can now go for hours without eating and do so much better. There are times still when I get a little wonky. And I do have to plan ahead for trips. I will scope out the restaurants that are best for my needs and, depending with whom I travel, try to find places where we can all enjoy a tasty meal. I will make reservations ahead of time if I can and mention my dietary restrictions.

It's not perfect. I still learn. Take my last trip to Italy with my husband. He so lovingly planned all the flights. I did the hotels, scoped out the restaurants, and brought travel snacks. We had a fabulous time. Then came the ride home. Meal-wise, I was ill-prepared. Two hours in the airport, then a nine-hour daytime flight. I thought, "Oh, I'll just fast. No problem." But it was a problem. I got really hungry and felt a bit wonky. So I ate the airplane food. Chicken and rice. How bad could it be? Apparently, delirium had set in. The food wasn't labelled gluten-free, so what should I have expected? Within hours of eating it, wowza. I think it's what you call a cytokine storm. I slept for three days, and when I wasn't sleeping, I was taking anything, anything to try to quench the snotty, achy mess I was in. My gut hurt for a month after that. I was irritable, and so were my bowels. Stupid. And I know better.

Thank goodness, my mood and energy are much more stable now that I've retrained my insulin sensitivity with diet, recognized food sensitivity, reset my microbiome, and gone through a period of fasting. You can do the same. But it's better to do so in a stable environment. Maybe not while travelling. It's always good to have some food security, just in case.

Fear impacts your microbiome.

I had to learn better strategies to combat it, or I would never get better.

When I am afraid, I imagine dressing myself in a full armour of protection. It comes with a belt of truth, a moral compass, a shield of faith to extinguish the flaming arrows of my opposition, a helmet of salvation, and shoes that help me walk with kindness and compassion. It is a lovely weave. In it, I deeply breathe in calm. I exhale slowly. Then I put together my plan of action from the most neutral place.

Fear comes in everyday packages. So does courage.

DENISE'S STORY

You must first neutralize negative emotions. Then you can turn them into love. This isn't always simple. Emotions get tangled up from time to time. Well, most of the time! Denise could attest to this.

You have to understand what kind of person Denise is. She is an all-loving, very nurturing, kind-hearted lady. For eighteen months, Denise held back her emotions around her sister. Over time, the relationship soured, and Denise felt a huge betrayal of trust. Once removed from the situation, Denise saw it was beyond her control to do anything about it. She kept swallowing her hurt, and it brewed inside of her. It is extremely painful when a love bond is broken. Other things in Denise's life added stress to her torment. She hadn't slept well, couldn't eat well, and due to stay-at-home restrictions from the government wasn't able to visit her parents and grandchildren. She felt very isolated with her feelings. She couldn't care for those she loved. She felt she needed to hush her emotions and be strong for her husband. The situation was unfathomable to her immediate family.

One day, Denise's husband was on the phone with her sister.

Something pulled the trigger for Denise. She lost it. All that hurt had brewed long enough and anger mounted. She screamed and yelled and cried and swore like crazy. Very out of character for Denise. Later, she felt anxious and guilty and panic set in. "What just happened?" she asked herself. "That wasn't even me who did and said all that." She shook like a leaf while on the phone with me, shocked that she could be so vicious and spiteful with her words. Now, in remorse, she admits she would never wish harm on anyone, but she feels lost.

When we don't express our hurt, it eventually brews into full-fledged anger. Anger that is suppressed is content under pressure. Shake it, and it will explode everywhere. I used the analogy of vomit with Denise. She had just thrown up all the anger and hurt she'd been holding in for months and months. If you've ever vomited, you know that once it starts, it cannot be stopped. It is stinky. It is messy. It tastes awful, and the acid lingers in your mouth for quite some time afterwards. It empties you. It is your body's way of forcing a fast exit for something that could be harmful. Emotions coming out can be very visceral. They come from the gut. Once you release the valve, there's no going back.

Once you are emptied out, you look at what you just did or said, and you may feel shame and guilt. That is what happened to Denise. Because she is genuinely a kind and loving soul, the anger was very difficult for her to experience. It was overwhelming. So we worked through the legitimate factors in her feelings. She needs to feel her feelings. Feelings need to be acknowledged. They do not need to be put in control. It was difficult for her to admit she was angry. However, this is what happens when we bottle up hurt. Eventually, it has to get out, or it can erode the soul. For Denise, now that's it out, it's out. It wasn't pretty. No. It wasn't nice either. But it's done. Now time to take out the mop and clean up the mess. Take some time to realize that it is out of you and that there still may be bits you missed cleaning up. There's some on the cupboard. How did it get halfway up the wall? Clean it up. Freshen yourself up, too. Have a bath with a cup of Epsom salts and a whole box of baking soda. It will help you neutralize. Denise said that helped. Forty-five minutes in the tub gave her time to be quiet and reflect. Although her feelings were justified and it felt better to acknowledge that they were, she was also concerned about putting anger out there. She didn't want any harm to come to anyone. That's fair. It's worthy, too.

Once you tell someone why you are angry with them, let it go. Figure out ways to release them from your anger. That's forgiveness. Forgiveness is not saying what they did was right. It's just saying you will not continue to allow them to hurt you with your anger. Now that the emotional bucket is emptied out, it is important to fill the void with good stuff. Otherwise, the bad stuff might rush back in. You have to love yourself after things like this. Lots and lots of love. Love will help you digest the world around you.

AMANDA'S STORY

Amanda came to see me because she was chronically ill. She'd used up all her sick days, and now her time off had eaten up all her vacation. She couldn't figure it out. We tested for the obvious things, felt around her belly to let it do the talking, boosted her immune status, and made some headway. Her digestion was off. We worked on her gut. Still, she noticed every time she was upset about work, she got sick. Sharp pain in the abdomen was her biggest symptom. She'd be home in bed, feeling like she had the flu, and having swings from diarrhea to difficult-to-pass stools all day. Eventually, we nailed down the timeline. This would happen whenever she feared she had disappointed her boss. Amanda worked so hard to be a good employee, work diligently, and look after her customers. Her boss had her own personal and emotional regulation issues. She often approached Amanda with suppressed anger. Amanda, unknowingly, picked up on the anger and frustration from her boss and internalized it in her gut. Most physicians would just chalk this up to anxiety and irritable bowel syndrome (IBS). No matter how you frame it, Amanda felt a direct stab into her gut from her boss. As we recognized the pattern, we began to build awareness and distinction of self from others. Amanda's fear was wrapped around disappointing her boss, but what she was truly experiencing was anger and frustration her boss was emitting. Her immune system acted in defence.

The realization that these emotions were not hers, but another's, helped Amanda tease apart the situation. When she stopped reacting to her boss's fleeting emotions and neutralized the reactionary fight-or-flight mode, Amanda felt more control over her own circumstances. She took ownership over her fear. When she felt compassion for her boss's inability to self-soothe, Amanda dispersed the negative hold her boss's feelings had on her. Still, there were times when the situation overwhelmed her. It was exhausting to continually work at separating, neutralizing, and letting go.

We all have an energy about us, like a fingerprint. It identifies us. We can tune into this. We transmit it like a wavelength. Like a receiver, we sense others'. We do this sensing through the gut.

Those who are universal givers of love often have an advanced sense of receiving. They are very sensitive people, heightened responders with very tuned-in solar plexus chakra. These people have a difficult time digesting their food *and* the world around them. They receive so much energy from their environment that they struggle to additionally digest food.

Those who are immature in their soul are immature in exercising the power of their solar (or is it soul-are?) plexus. They broadcast raw energy haphazardly. Pushing out, pushing out, pushing out their energy to the world. Look at me, look at me, look at me. They take up so much bandwidth! Take. Take. Take. The takers never find what they are looking for because they have yet to develop their receiving station. They ignore their gut sense. They have a terrible time receiving any kind of love or compassion. The gut must first sense before the heart can feel. They really have a heyday with those who are good givers, people who are well tuned into their sensations but lack the discernment, boundaries, or standards and criteria to tell when it is not appropriate to give. Interesting that emotions have boundaries, and the gut does, too! Does one reflect the other? Perhaps.

Those with an underdeveloped solar plexus fight with food in their own specific ways. Either they eat too much, trying to receive through their food what they cannot get from other aspects of the outside world, or they eat the wrong kinds of food to get the "hit" they crave. Sugar, gluten, and gluteomorphins are prime examples.

We know that if the solar plexus is imbalanced (whether excessive or deficient) or unevolved, it will lead to digestive disorders, eating disorders, ulcers, or problems in the liver, pancreas, stomach, and gallbladder. If this is you, you need grounding and emotional warmth as a part of your healing protocol. Animals are a great source of emotional warmth. If you don't have one or can't afford one, go to your local animal shelter and see about volunteering. I've sent all sorts of people out to be bunny cuddlers, dog walkers, or local sanctuary help. It can be very rewarding.

To ground, we look to the root chakra, the base of the spine. If the energy here is deficient, you will disconnect from your body altogether, be up in your head too much, or not even be emotionally present. At times, we are so in our heads that our bodies lie in neglect. If you have excessive energy in your root chakra, you may hoard or overeat. Balance yourself by walking barefoot in the morning grass, hiking along a natural path or trail, simply lying on the ground, or having a picnic outside. Swimming in the ocean or sea is remarkable. All the minerals in the saltwater are infinitely healing.

Sitting and breathing quietly helps you simply bring awareness to your breath, honouring it. Appreciation is a tool for focus as well. Find three things you are thankful for every day. At least three. If you can find more, then continue to count your blessings!

Amanda worked through the process of grounding, breath, and solar plexus awareness.

Two years later, she built enough confidence to move into a more senior role at another company. Her former boss never really changed. It was time for Amanda to move on and rise to other opportunities. Her learning with her previous employer was done. Now Amanda is more attuned to her sensitivities to others' energy, and we work to help her strengthen her own inner voice. She freed herself from the unevolved emotions of her previous boss. Working on her own truth, Amanda is wise when she feels pangs in her gut. She listens and honours and brings love to how and what she feels.

You ask, "Can a bad day make me sick?" Yes, it can, if the stress is chronic or you lack the skills to deal with it. A bad day could also ignite your fight-or-flight response to make you stronger. The old adage "What doesn't kill us makes us stronger" is true if the body adapts and has reprieve to rest and restore. Many bad days in a row, over an extended length of time can weaken the immune defence and increase risk of illness. See how Amanda overcame this? You can, too. It takes time. We worked physically, emotionally, cognitively, and spiritually. Amanda, like you and me, continues to evolve. Through her journey, it is critical to continue to support her immune system. For her, a probiotic, B complex, and blend of seven different immune mushrooms and some zinc at times does the trick. Keep your immune system strong, keep your microbiome strong, keep your defence strong.

IMMUNE SYSTEM AS YOUR DEFENCE: THE GOOD FIGHT

It is our natural primitive response to defend ourselves. We need armour. Without it, we wouldn't survive. Simple. As a child, you depend on your parents to keep you safe from harm. Ask any mother if she ever heard noises in the night before her child was born. It's unlikely she did. However, once an infant or dependent requires your care, from the dead of sleep, you can hear even a sigh from the other room. We are wired to defend. As you grow, you learn to watch out for danger. You learn to take care of yourself. As you learn to distinguish safe from unsafe, so does your immune system. Your nervous system and your immune system constantly survey information from the environment. Both consciously and unconsciously, they are primed to detect danger.

When the body starts attacking itself, that's autoimmune disease. Generally, if you have an autoimmune disease, your nervous system is very primed. You, my dear, have been "on the watch" for way too long. Just like your immune system is overreacting, so too is your nervous system. Warfare takes its toll on the surrounding territory.

Autoimmune disease often starts with a breach in the gastrointestinal lining. Leaky gut, lack of boundaries, oversurveillance to counter what seeps through the wall. The gut lining, like a castle wall that is only one brick thick, is breached. There is a hole in the wall, and dangerous invaders can creep through. Particles that should stay in the gut lumen (your digestive track tube) are now floating around inside of you. The immune troops outside the castle wall (your gut) let you down, and now there are invaders in your castle.

Think of this both in terms of physical and emotional layers. Your gut is a wall. You set up emotional barriers, which are also like walls. Sooner or later, your personality reflects these walls. This means you likely jump at the quietest noise, attack in conversations, and have very disrupted sleep. In this state, it is very difficult to trust anyone. When I was there, I couldn't even trust myself. It is truly a state of unrest. Imagine you have a camera, and you zoom in and out. What's happening on the cellular level is also happening on the interpersonal level.

Please bear with me on a few details for a moment as I try to sum up the importance of gut health, your immune system, and your longevity. I want to really drive home how the immune system directs behaviour and another way the gut is implicated in anxiety and depression.

The immune system is complex in one way, but easy to understand if you think of it as your personal security system. It all has to do with the chemical messengers that deliver messages from cell to cell. What else would they do, right?

What is interesting is the word "messenger" suggests goodness and is often used to refer to someone who offers comfort and aid to others in times of trouble. Some might call this an angel. Let's imagine it this way.

There are several types of "angels" in your body. Scientists call them cytokines. What's important overall is that these angels can be traced. Tracked. Measured. Like they are on a GPS.

Over the course of many years and studies and observations, scientists have found that abnormal levels of different kinds of these "angels," whether too many for too long or too many of one kind versus another, are evident in patients with many chronic diseases and digestive and mood disorders. Now, if you have a lot of angels running around trying to tell different parts of your body that danger is lurking, are they the bad guys? No. Don't shoot the messenger, right? Having just the right balance of angels is pretty helpful. But when there is danger lurking, they increase in numbers to sound the alarm.

Depression, anxiety, schizophrenia, Alzheimer's, insomnia, and leaky gut are good reasons for alarm. These are chronic sources of inflammation. Why inflammation? Is it altogether bad? No. Short term, inflammation is very helpful. It is there to help take away the garbage from a site of trauma, infection, or injury. Like a first responder.

When there is an overload of food sensitivity, unprocessed emotional chemicals, toxins, or viral, bacterial, fungal, or parasitic load, the first responders can't keep up with the chronic activation. It's too much.

On the contrary, think of how it feels to run free in an open park. All lush, mowed, with flowers growing. Clear streams running fluidly. Freedom. Ease of movement. You can run with your arms open wide and breathe fresh air, pain-free. This is a clean lymphatic system. It can keep up with the demands and provides a well of nourishment.

The onset of digestive and gastrointestinal issues often begins in times when you take on information that is beyond your capacity to digest. Or you eat too many of the wrong foods that are difficult to digest. Inflammation happens especially in times of grief, abuse, or other major negative life events. Instead of taking what you need and letting go of the rest, you keep adding to a bucket without a release valve.

Thus, inflammation clogs you up. Think about it this way: If you are trying to move through a room and it is full of stuff, how annoying is it to get through as you are bumping into everything? You feel stuck, you can't get through, and ouch, you hit something. This can make you feel frustrated. Well, your lymphatics (immune system inside the body) work similarly. Lymph is your sewer system, so to speak. It delivers white blood cells to fight infection and takes away debris from the war zone of infection.

If there is a bunch of garbage floating around your insides and your lymphatics can't keep up with it, they get sluggish and dirty. Just like the streets after a St. Paddy Day's party at the local college. A mess. Garbage, puke, junk, all left behind. Some of it bagged up, some cluttered in the gutter. This is your lymphatic system hard at work. It just can't keep up with all the big parties going on. Clutter in your gutter? You are going to feel sluggish, anxious, maybe even depressed. This is when your cells give off a danger response, and the chemical messengers try to tell all the other cells to prepare for battle. Your angels are overwhelmed trying to protect you.

If you are overrun with angels and all these obstacles to health, you will eventually come to a standstill. It is then difficult for you to experience pleasure and you can even start to feel helpless.[145] They are sounding so many alarms that you literally become immobilized with fear. Freeze mode. Ever felt that way? I think most of the world does while they stay locked up at home through a pandemic. Prime example. Not a helpful state to be in when it's time to go back out again and run the risk of a viral attack and cytokine storm.

Your digestion shuts down in fight-or-flight mode. Your body releases cortisol so you can get sugars into the bloodstream and

145 Vogelzangs, N., de Jonge, P., Smit, J. H., Bahn, S., & Penninx, B. W. (2016). Cytokine production capacity in depression and anxiety. *Translational Psychiatry*, 6(5), e825. https://doi.org/10.1038/tp.2016.92

flee to safety, blood flow goes to the extremities to allow your muscles to act, and your heart rate increases. This is no time for processing food.

It perplexes me. How can it be that we have lived in human bodies for thousands of years and still do not fully grasp how our physical, emotional, cognitive, and spiritual layers are knit together?

What wisdom we have lost.

If you want to digest, you need rest, a break, and reprieve to keep up with the demands. You cannot operate 24/7 for long. Every period of intense activity must be followed by a period of intense rest. For every yin there is a yang. Vice versa. Balance. Like when we talked about biorhythms—you need day and night.

You might feel a little uneasy right now. That's allowed. Sometimes when you are so used to cortisol, adrenaline, and fear pumping through your body, the mere idea that you may be better resting can make you edgy, almost as if you are addicted to stress.

Pause and give thanks to your gut and your amazing immune system. Recognize a time when you displayed courage to face a fear, regardless of the outcome. Place awareness around your navel area. Maybe rest your hands on it for a few minutes and just be. When you are ready, come back, and we'll see if there is any need for faith in your forecast.

10

CORE STRENGTH

Here's what you'll learn in this chapter:

- Why boundaries are important in your gut and in life
- The gut-heart-mind connection
- The power of breath and how to use it

THE HEALING IS WITHIN

"You don't have a soul. You are a soul. You have a body."

—C. S. LEWIS

I never forget the time in my life when everything seemed to be falling apart on the outside. Faith was something that was very new to me. Up to then, I'd trained well in the gym and had abs of steel. With gymnastics in childhood and competitive fitness in my teens, this was a natural body state for me. There's even a picture of me when I was about 8 or 9, jumping off these gigantic sand hills near the shores of Lake Erie. You could see the six-pack under the swimsuit. Exercise is a way of life for me. I love to do it first thing in the morning so I can get a hold of the day before it gets hold of me. Exercise and movement are critical to good health. But in my late twenties and early thirties, as my gut health deteriorated, what I sought after most was a different kind of core strength. I asked my spiritual leader, "How can I build strength from the inside out?" I wanted core strength that would give me a rock on which to build my life. In times when I felt I could easily collapse in on myself, it was what I sought out strongly without even knowing what it was all about.

I recognized I was missing something. Life, driven by my own will, wasn't working out so well for me. Not in my job, my marriage, or family relationships. As I prayed, for first time in my life, I got to know our creator. Our universal source of energy and love. There is no difference in the body and spirit you live in as it is described by a Western or Eastern practitioner. Same body. Same mind. Same Spirit. All that differs is how it is described or observed. Like the blind men and the elephant. All feeling different parts of the elephant, describing what they sense. It feels different to each of them, but it's still an elephant.

Maybe the elephant in the room, the thing we are not talking about, is the element of the creator that lives within us. Maybe, just maybe, harmony with the Holy Spirit is the final layer of healing. How so? There is no science to this. Yet. But what if the lack of divine nature living within us is what keeps our microbiome from healing itself?

We must live in harmony with the microbes in our gut. They serve us. We serve them. This is what is called a symbiotic relationship.

Our goal is not to control them. Most digestion is out of our control. I still want to control so many aspects of my life. In reality, I can control only about 20 percent of it.

What we need to do is provide the playing ground for the microbes to thrive so we, too, can thrive. It is essential. Could it be that Spirit is like a conductor in our body? We must find better ways to resonate with its vibration.

What helps you digest the world in which you live so that it does not digest you?

I used to think I needed to set better boundaries. I am really terrible with boundaries. I am better than I once was but not as good as I think I could be. I think it's because it is easier for me to care for someone than not to care. My heart is willing to pour itself out. This is not always healthy. It doesn't help when you spend a lot of time around someone who constantly oversteps their boundaries and doesn't respect yours. It is an exhausting experience.

It made more sense to me when a spiritual leader told me women, innately, do not set boundaries. They set standards and criteria. Reflect on this for yourself.

After I took a couple of days to absorb this into my being, I feel my standards are truth and light. I have to feel you seek the truth and light before I can let you into my space. It's not a wall you have to climb. Your intentions and what you carry in your heart are what matter to me. Also, remember, there are male and female aspects to us all. In some situations, it makes sense to set boundaries. In others, standards and criteria are the better fit.

You strive to look after the body in so many important ways. The drugs you take, the sleep you get, your environment, your water, your food packaging, genetics, your age, alcohol, meal timing, food quality, and quantity can all affect your microbiome. When you are physically, cognitively, and emotionally fit, you think, speak, and hear clearly. Cognition is a reflection of how well the physical and emotional layers tie together. Your immune system, nervous system, and endocrine systems are defined by the long word *psychoneuro-immunology*. These are all layers in the onion.

THE HEART-GUT CONNECTION

The ancients believed the small intestine and the heart were paired as yin-and-yang organs. We know what passes from the gastrointestinal tract into the bloodstream will eventually flow through the heart. The small intestine lends decision-making capacity for issues of the heart, and the heart gives mental clarity and integration to the small intestine. But what does this mean in Western ideology of physical health? Simply put, your heart has to be in the right place emotionally for your digestion to be right. Work on the heart, and it will help the food go down.

Clearly, the gut picks up on what goes on in the environment and makes emotional chemicals. Then the heart feels the results. When you receive difficult news, sometimes it feels like too much to digest. Otherwise, why would one feel like vomiting after getting bad news? For example, when my first husband told me he didn't love me and loved someone else, I ran straight for the bathroom and dry heaved for what seemed to be hours. My heart hurt, and I could barely eat for weeks. I had trouble digesting the news. My gut was sensing so much around me and the energy backed up because my heart was overwhelmed with trying to feel the swell of emotions. Since my heart couldn't process what had happened, there was no way my mind could make sense of it. It is important that the heart feels through emotions to prevent a digestive block.

Sadness and depression can be related to heart health. Another way to look at the gut-heart-brain connection: intestinal permeability (leaky gut) can increase inflammatory factors in the bloodstream, which lead to unstable plaque in your arteries (cardiovascular disease) and inflammation in the brain (depression).

Yes, unstable plaque can be the start of a cascade of clots, embolisms, and insulin dysregulation. However, in the famous Framingham research that launched the campaign for statin drugs against cholesterol, heart rate variability (HRV), or beat-to-beat variation of the heart, was more of a determinant of health than LDL cholesterol levels. As you learned with George's story, HRV is the cornerstone to the HeartMath® breathing techniques.

BREATH

What is the mystery that breathes life into you? Breath is the first gift of life. You take it everywhere you go. Spirit, a word from Latin origin, literally means breath. It is the animating, sensitive, vital principle of being. It is not mystical or supernatural. Breath is what keeps you alive. It separates life from death.

Think about it. We are not ever truly still. Thanks to our breath, we are in constant motion. Emotional regulation, spiritual connection, and gut health are intricately connected.

The core of your being is where your soul and spirit connect. You have a soul? No. As C. S. Lewis clarified, you *are* a soul; you have a body. Your breath connects your soul with the Spirit. As you explore the Spirit and how to use your breath, it becomes one with you. It serves you in the best way: to sustain life.

Ever notice life gives you lessons? If you learn, you move on to a new lesson. If you don't, you stay stuck and keep running into the same situation in different parts of your life. Same crap, different pile. Pay attention. When you get stuck in this negative realm of emotions, it prolongs the release of cortisol. As you learned earlier, cortisol is very helpful in the short term. It mounts a response (fight! run!) that could save your life. You get stronger from the experience when you learn from it and move on from it. Sometimes life throws more at you than you are prepared to handle. It can be one big thing, but more often it is a series of events, one after the other, and it is easy to get stuck in the weeds. When this happens, cortisol surges from your adrenal glands. Your hypothalamus tries to respond and counteracts the surge in various ways. You get headaches, blood pressure rises, and hormone imbalances. The microbiome gets disrupted, and your immune system is compromised.

As you stay in a realm of negativity, chemicals are released that damage the cells in your body. Literally, your cell walls begin to harden and become less flexible—as do you. We must digest emotions separately from our food. Just as we have physical enzymes that break down food, we have physical enzymes that break down our emotions. The chemicals that cause emotions are called catecholamines—epinephrine, norepinephrine or adrenaline, and cortisol. If you are busy "digesting" an event emotionally, you will have difficulty digesting your food at the same time. Take time to invest in the skills you need to deal with stress.

No one else can do it for you. Not even me. I can give you supplements to help correct nutritional deficiencies. I can run tests to give you feedback on what's going on in your body. I can provide you with education and give you ideas for what to do. But I cannot connect your soul with the Spirit because I cannot breathe for you. You must breathe for yourself. Practice. Time. Dedication. Focus.

Each beat-to-beat variation of the heart rate is tied to a signature emotion. When you are feeling down, the rhythm is much different from when you feel agitated or anxious. The intensity of your emotions depends on the height of your nervous system's response. Give you something you've dealt with well a hundred times before, or a sense of loss, and the amplitude is pretty low. Put you in a situation that is something new or a threat, and you get "amped" up. The neurotransmitters released in the body are responsible for turning the dial up or down. A higher amplitude can be the result of either anxiety or excitement. It all depends on how you look at the new situation.

The heart is an amazing organ. It is a muscle. Like any muscle, it has memory and can be trained. Think of an athlete. Maybe you are one. Did you ride a bike, dance, skate, shoot hoops, or play on a team? Think of a musician. Maybe you are one. What is it like to learn a new routine, a new play on the field, or a new song? At first, you are a little clunky. Uncoordinated. You have to break down the new piece into smaller pieces to get it right. Then once you've done that, you can put it all together. As you practice, it becomes second nature. Then, even years later, you just need to play the first few notes, or sit on that bike and start peddling. Voilà! Your muscle memory takes over, and away you go again. Same goes for the heart. You can train it down a path that is positive or negative. It much prefers the positive. Learn the HeartMath® (heartmath.org) skills in four to five weekly sessions with a HeartMath® Certified Professional. In between sessions, practice what you learn for five to fifteen minutes a day, and you will be able to shift yourself from the negative depleting emotions to ones of calm energy, with the focus, concentration, grace, and flow of an athlete or musician. Soon, your positive energy will impact others and your interactions will go much more smoothly. Remember, the mind thinks, the gut senses, and the heart, well, it feels everything.

How does this work? The heart is more than a muscle. It also generates pulse waves through the bloodstream, gives off neurotransmitters if it is in distress, and emits electromagnetic waves detectable up to 3 feet from the body. Arguably, the waves permeate beyond this and we lack the equipment to properly measure it. You know when you are in a room of people? At an event or cocktail party or something. You can be engaged in conversation with someone with your back turned to the door. People can come and go from that door. However, with some unique individuals, you can sense their presence as they enter the room without even turning around to see them. It can be a positive or negative feeling you sense. The gut senses. You turn around and notice. A charismatic individual often possesses this ability to emit strong positive electromagnetic waves. You, too, can learn this. Imagine having these positive waves swimming around in your body at your command. You can create them.

When you are calm, your digestion calms. The heart has to be there to help the gut. Use your breath and focussed intention to help calm your nervous system and hormones. All of this provides space for your soul and the Spirit to connect.

I have taught this for a number of years now. See if it works for you. I also like the idea of breathing through the gut centre. The solar plexus. Read on to see what I mean. There are many ways to use your breath. It's a tool you take everywhere with you.

TIME BETWEEN BREATHS

Transcend time and space in the subtle moment between your inhale and exhale. Pause for a moment to try this technique. Breathe in and out for five breaths: in through your nose and out through your mouth. With each breath, exhale longer and longer. You will naturally inhale longer as your lung capacity strengthens. Keep the breath slow and gentle. Try to breathe out long after you think you may be done. As you create a rhythm, close your eyes. In the time between in and out, as you transition from inhale to exhale, notice the pause. Continue the practice for as long as you like. The stillness, the pause, and the time between breaths help calm the nervous system. Calm in the nervous system will help create calm in the gut.

BREATH OF FIRE

Ever step into a cold shower? Try it. What happens to your breath? It goes right from your navel in quick rhythmic ins and outs. This is the start of the idea of the breath of fire. Stand in the cold shower for a couple of minutes while doing this kind of breath, and it will warm you up! It will also fire up your energy, release toxins, expand lung capacity, and increase vitality.

The breath of fire is sometimes called the detox breath. It is meant to go a little faster, a big breath in and out through your nose. It is very liberating for the lymphatic system and helps drain out toxins. It supports the immune system and ultimately digestion. Practice it five minutes a day, and in a few days you will truly feel stronger and clearer.

Try it. First, push your navel out as you draw in your breath. Second, on the exhale, draw your navel back to your spine. Try it slowly. Do your best to equalize the inhale with the exhale. Start slow. Like an old steam engine pulling out of the station. Breathe in and out, through the nose. Expel the moisture in your nose with a soft force, like you are trying to blow out a candle. Inhale with equal force. Then pick up the pace. If it helps, you can place a hand on the belly to feel it go out when you breathe in. As you find a rhythm, pump the breaths a little faster. Imagine someone putting pressure on your belly and lower back to squeeze the air out. The power comes from the navel, the area of the solar plexus. The solar plexus is a nerve centre of energy that not only connects you to yourself but also the universal energy. This makes sense as the navel is the remnants of the umbilical cord where, while in the womb, you were once attached to your mother. It is where emotional joins the mental in understanding and the primal place of connection to feminine, nurturing energy. It is where you sense the world around you. The gut senses.

Begin your practice with one-minute sessions. Then increase the duration to two to three minutes. Work your way up to ten minutes. The body should remain relaxed through the cycle. If you feel dizzy or lightheaded, you may be inhaling more than you are exhaling. If you feel weak, distracted, or depressed, you may be exhaling more than you are inhaling. As it becomes rhythmic, speed it up. Full steam ahead!

The solar plexus area uplifts your personal sense of power; governs your gut feelings, digestion, metabolism, and emotions; and influences the immune, nervous, and muscular systems. For more information, look into Kundalini yoga or visit www.3HO.org.

This technique is not recommended for pregnant or menstruating females.

WIM HOF'S BREATHING TECHNIQUE

A world record holder in icy realms, Wim Hof, "the Iceman," teaches how breath and a focussed mindset can alter the state of nervous system. The Wim Hof Breath (WHB) technique involves inhalation with force and exhalation as it naturally follows. By not breathing out entirely, you cause residual air to build in the lungs. The principle chemistry of breath is oxygen in, carbon dioxide out. With the WHB technique, after forty-five minutes of practice, the oxygen you draw into the body is doubled. You exhale less carbon dioxide, and the pH of the blood gets more alkaline (less acidic). This prevents the production of lactic acid, the chemical that makes your muscles ache after a hard workout. It also overrides the autonomic nervous system and strengthens the immune system, both of which are related to gut health.[146]

146 Muzik, O., Reilly, K. T., & Diwadkar, V. A. (2018). "Brain over body": A study on the willful regulation of autonomic function during cold exposure. *NeuroImage*, 172, 632–641. https://doi.org/10.1016/j. neuroimage.2018.01.067

See https://www.wimhofmethod.com/science for more information.

UJJAYI BREATH

Pronounced *oo-jai*, this is sometimes referred to as the victorious breath. Think of your vagal nerve as well. Victory for the vagal nerve. Jumping for joy. Ujjayi. It will help balance your nervous system. Since we need the vagal nerve to balance before we can properly digest our food, this is critically important.

Start by sitting comfortably in a chair, feet flat on the ground. Breathe in deeply through the nose, and imagine the muscles at the top of your windpipe are contracting. You will hear and feel your breath at the back of your throat when you do this.

Next, breathe out as slowly as possible, pushing the air gently out of your nose. Close off the mouth by pushing the back of your tongue against the roof of your mouth.

Breathe in and out like this six times, then take six normal breaths. Repeat for a few minutes.

COOLING BREATH

Chill out. Sometimes you need a way to dispel heat from the body. Anger, irritation, inflammation? All heat. Remember, it's about balance. Too much heat, cool it off. If you are cold or feeling chilled, don't do this!

Sit comfortably with your feet flat on the floor and hands gently in your lap. As you close your eyes to tune out the distractions, focus in on your breath. In. Out.

Next, stick your tongue out gently so it rests on your lower lip. Make an O out of your lips and curl your tongue into a tube, like you are making a straw out of it. Breathe slowly in and out. Feel the cool air draw through your tongue tube. Breathe deeply, draw the air through the tongue tube, and imagine the tube reaching down deep into your belly. Fill it up. Let it out. As you breathe in and out like this, you may feel a cooling sensation up and down your body. It's like you are providing a gentle breeze inside of it. Continue for a few minutes or until you feel the irritation or anger dissipate.

HUM OR SING

When you hum or sing, you are actually breathing out. Take a breath in, then allow a sound to come out by humming or singing. The vibration of the sound is an added benefit to the vagus nerve activation and therefore is very healing for the gut.

As shown through extensive research from HeartMath®, connection with breath naturally alters the electromagnetic waves, or vibrations, in your body. Vibrational therapy has anti-inflammatory and disease-reversing effects on your health and that of your microbiome.[147] Think of the waves discussed in the previous chapter and how the microbiome attunes to those. A vibration is made of waves! I propose that tuning into a more

---

147 Yu, J. C., Hale, V. L., Khodadadi, H., & Baban, B. (2019). Whole body vibration-induced omental macrophage polarization and fecal microbiome modification in a murine model. *International Journal of Molecular Sciences*, 20(13), 3125. https://doi.org/10.3390/ijms20133125

positive frequency encourages both our human cells and the trillions of microbes in our gut to resonate and work harmoniously.

Allow your breath and your focussed attention to create a vibrational force that resonates within you. If you have difficulty engaging, remember a time when you felt most at home in your body. Or sing your favourite song out loud in the car or the shower. Lean into feeling open, soft, and expansive.

When you are ready, come on back. We'll further explore how the gut connects to your soul.

WELCOME HOME

Here's what you'll learn in this chapter:

- Heal from the inside out
- Appreciate how you are knit together
- Allow the rise of the feminine, subdue the masculine, engage digestion
- The connection between your gut and your soul

The layers of your onion are fully exposed. You worked through the physical, the emotional, and cognitive layers. You reached your inner onion, your true spiritual core, and now you can work on healing the body from the inside out. The healing is truly within.

Your body is a miracle and a profound mystery. However much you have learned, there is so much more to discover. Your continued health relies not on separating body, mind, and spirit, but understanding and appreciating how they might be knit together.

MAXWELL'S STORY

Maxwell comes to me with tremor issues. Single and 50, he is embarrassed to go out on a date with anyone because he can't even pick up a fork without shaking. All tests come back negative for anything related to Parkinson's or any other measurable neurological condition. He has a family history of anxiety and a personal history of eating next-to-no vegetables. He exercises regularly to balance his desk job as a database code writer. After two years of dietary coaching and supplementing, we peel back all the physical layers of the onion. He keeps weekly diet and activity diaries. Slowly, week by week, he makes more conscious eating decisions. Initially, he supplements with a ton of magnesium, zinc, N-acetyl-cysteine, vitamin C, and even does SAMe for a while. Emotionally, Maxwell fixates on the sexual side of a relationship with women. He is tuned only into his masculine energy and has no idea how to manage his softer emotional side. He treats encounters with women as if they are an unattainable object he does not deserve. I see it as a lack of connection with his own heart, void in Spirit. I have to meet Maxwell where he is at. The physical plane. I have no idea how far I can lead him, or how long he will stick around for guidance. He perseveres. I dose NatSulph homeopathic 200 C on occasion. After eighteen months, his cognitive layer starts to peel. He begins reading books. Remember, cognition is the process of acquiring knowledge and understanding through thought, experience, and the senses. All the while, I keep seeing visions of what would be his wedding day. Sitting far back in the aisle, observing how far he'd come. How a sterile soul could be revived. To find love first for his own soul, then the opportunity to share that with another.

Through six months of cognitive work, we continue nutritional counsel and tremor monitoring and dig deeper into the senses. We begin the HeartMath® program in session in the clinic. He likes to see the biofeedback of the rhythms of his heart. But he cannot recall a time of love, care, or appreciation for someone or something. He has difficulty connecting with his heart. There is a block. We focus on breath. Counting breaths. Slowing the breath. Deepening the breath. We dive into past experiences that stick out in his memory. We tease them apart. Three weeks go by, then a month, then another month. Maxwell finds his tremor is almost gone. He lets go of things from his past. He learns to accept himself. To be himself. To be okay being himself. He puts lettuce in his chicken and rice wrap. He puts broccoli and kale in his omelet. He learns how to cook a sweet potato. He eats avocados and caesar salad. Green is the energetic colour of the heart centre.

Last Saturday, Maxwell wakes up and says it feels like Christmas. There is JOY in his heart. He can feel the breath come and go from his heart. He feels his heart. He feels free. Free from the past. Free from anxiety. Free to move forward. Let go of negativity. I ask him to tell me more about it. He says he believes in evolution. A giraffe has a long neck, having evolved to eat the leaves on the higher branches. Maxwell doesn't want to go to Church. He wonders what this Spirit of joy is that he feels when he breathes into his heart. He cries. I ask why it has to be one or the other. Evolution or faith? Can they not be one and the same?

No work of art is ever finished. This is creation. It takes a while to create a masterpiece. Like the world evolved, so too is Maxwell a creation. A work of art. Never finished. Still evolving. We have peeled the physical, emotional, cognitive layers of his onion. We made it to the centre, the core, the spiritual layer. But just as soon as we bask in the glorious light at this level, it grows outward, too; we grow deeper, layers continue to evolve from the inside out. What once was in the centre moves outward, spiritual layers grow out to affect the cognitive layer, the emotional layer, then the physical layer. Just as the food we eat nourishes the entire body, as we feed the soul and invite the Spirit in, it renews us from the inside out. The healing truly is within. Shining its bright light out. We must continue to shed the external peel to allow the inside to grow. We must continue to breathe, to renew, to invite the Divine Spirit and light into our hearts. It will encourage our soul. It will renew.

Writing the first part of the book was a linear, straightforward, logical exercise; a transaction; easy to lay out, control the outcome, and support my claims to knowledge with evidence-based medical research. This is masculine energy at its best. You have masculine energy. You also have feminine energy. A yang and a yin. As I come closer to the second part, resistance builds in me. Sleep is disrupted. Dreams are intense. My body feels like it is detoxing. Fatigue in the day. Burning through my veins. Mild headache that comes and goes. Thirsty. Craving salt. Lots of full bowel movements. No tolerance for caffeine or alcohol.

Why is this? All the while, the sacred feminine, the Divine keeps coming up in my thoughts. I woke up last night to a flurry of random connections. What is masculine? It is the chalice, the point, the penis, the control, the power over things? What have we done in this past half century? Aspired to the science, the power, the knowledge, the evidenced-based medicine, the control, the feminist movement, the certainties, the consistent, reliable protection of being on guard. While we are on guard as a collective, we engage (continually) the sympathetic nervous system. When the sympathetic nervous system is engaged, guess what disengages? Digestion.

STUCK IN OVERDRIVE

I checked in with Marillia yesterday to remind her of her appointment. She said, "You know, I am not sure what we will talk about. I think in all, I was just tired. And now, with a month off work, I have had lots of rest and feel so much better."

Marillia is not alone. Our entire society has been on overdrive. As you and I engage our sympathetic nervous system, our digestion shuts down. Our whole society has shut down its digestive capacity, both for food and for those around us. This makes one irritable. You can't continually run on overdrive. The yang energy will consume the yin energy. Over the past half century, we've lost connection with our environment, our earth, our food, ourselves, and our souls. Powered by distraction and striving for power over everything and anything, we have left wisdom behind. But even the Bible says wisdom is more valuable than gold: Proverbs 3:14–24, Proverbs 8:11, Proverbs 16:16, Job 28:17–19.

Years ago, I belonged to a women's workgroup that met for monthly lunches. When I was invited to join, I thought I would find comfort in company of like-minded business counterparts. I had left the role of senior sales executive for a large software enterprise behind, and after years of reeducation, I had donned the hat of a naturopathic doctor. My first career was very male-dominated, my second, very female-dominated. Many of the conversations around the table were about how to be equal in power to males in the workplace. How to fight for job placements after pregnancy leave. Break that glass ceiling. I thought to myself, "Really? This still exists?"

There was a ton of fear around child-rearing and loss of status. The group members' sense of community was strong with their female work colleagues, weak in their neighbourhoods and homes. They were afraid to embrace their sacred feminine nurturing qualities, like they had to leave those behind if they were to become successful. Let me share a secret with you. Feminine energy is estimated (by spiritual elders) to be 60x more intuitive than the masculine. This scares the kejeebers out of anyone with primarily male-oriented energy. This is likely why female-oriented people, and the female parts of ourselves, are suppressed. The male energy feels the loss of control, so it retaliates. When power and control over others are the dominant values in society, guess what happens? Right. Everyone wants the power and control.

"What's the opposite of this flurry? What is the opposite of power and control and dominance?" I ask myself. Control is very masculine. Yang. Outward energy. Motion. So what is the yin, the opposite of masculinity and control? Substance. Matter. Femininity. Surrender. What is surrender? What does that mean? It means to give up the fight. To work with, rather than against, the other. To power *under*, rather than over, someone else. To power under is to lift. To lift up our brothers and sisters. A womb holds, lifts, protects, provides covering. Shelter. Provides a lifeline of nourishment. When you are in a womb, you trust, without question, that everything you need is provided. It doesn't take a big leap of faith; early in our lives, it is the only experience we know.

I believe that as a society, we have fought long and hard. Our societal battle is as intense as the immune battle in our bodies. On both fronts, we have idolized the masculine qualities of power, force, and control. How could we not? We demand science-based evidence, proof, to make a point. Although these things are important, they need to be taken in context and balance with the wisdom passed on through generations: the innate knowing, the feminine intuitive capacity available to us all. We need this to guide our bodies and ourselves in the world around us.

LET YOUR GUARD DOWN

What happens now when you let your guard down, rest, rejuvenate?

You digest your food and the world around you.

All this, and I am still afraid to let my guard down. Are you? This tells me that I am not yet fully trusting in my faith. It also tells me why I may not be fully digesting my food or the world around me, even though I'd like to. Divine energy holds me up all this time, and still I cannot trust it? I am cool with hanging out with Jesus. I rather like him as a friend. I met him when life brought me to my knees, literally. I was separated, going through divorce, and making choices to move from the family home, exit from the business my former husband and I owned, and choose shared access to the children. My faith guided me through many decisions to move forward in my life. These experiences strengthened my faith, and not too long after, it was further strengthened when I was diagnosed with a tumour on my tailbone that had wrapped around all my intestines. (Strange thing that was.) I made it out alive, the tumour was not cancerous, and after a second surgery, I was on the mend. In it, however, I had to surrender how I looked at life.

But how is the heart that feels different from the gut that intuits? Ah. There is the difference. The heart feels everything we do. The gut senses, the heart feels, then the mind thinks. I must have tuned out my gut sense. I was afraid to honour this feminine counterpart. I, too, was on the wagon of power, control, science, proof, construct, organization, logic, data. Head knowledge. Easy to gain.

Wisdom, gut intuition, on the other hand, I'd suppressed all these years. Not that the information wasn't being picked up. Like a sponge, I absorb everything around me. I'd just neglected to set up boundaries, standards, and criteria. It was a free for all consuming me. My gut barrier was a sieve and so was my personal space.

In hindsight, I can see what happened. Through the breakdown of my first marriage, I no longer trusted my partner. It was even more difficult to trust myself and my choices. Then, going through the college of naturopathic medicine, where everything was about evidence-based research, I shut down the trust in my gut even further. Thus, I was not secure enough to trust my intuition, feeling always like I had to prove something, not only to others but to myself. Looking in book after book for what is never found in a book: my soul.

Oh, good Lord, what sits right now on my bedside table beside my Bible? A new age book on *Soul Love*.

We need to balance our masculine energy, which dominates society and our individual bodies, with more feminine nature and nurture. The pendulum need not shift to the opposite extreme. Simply return us back to centre so that we love, trust, and respect ourselves and others; so that quality of character comes first and foremost. Power under, not over, others.

My big question is, if you and I have done all the outward physical things to support gut health—worked through our emotional attachments to food, gotten good exercise, and supported healthy sleep habits—yet still have issues with our gut, will they, can they, be resolved through a close spiritual connection? This question drives me nuts, possibly because spiritual connection is so mysterious.

What exactly is a soul? A soul is the spiritual immortal substance or essence crafted by our great creator. It has an energy, which means it has a frequency. No energy is ever destroyed or created; it is only transformed into another state. That's physics. Universal laws of nature that never change. Easy to trust those.

Your gut is a place where physical energy of food transforms to physical energy in your body; it is also where you connect to the world around you and to the energy of higher beings. Your gut is the birthplace of etheric body—your primary essence or energy. Your primary essence is what some call the vis, which is Latin for power or force. In Chinese medicine, it's the qi, or circulating life force.

"Be not anxious, but trust."

—PHILIPPIANS 4:6-7

It is clear that an anxious, unrested soul is one disconnected from spiritual health. Anxiety is a wrinkle between an individual's soul and the heavenly Spirit. It also is a wrinkle in the gut, an imbalance in the microbiome. A vibration out of harmony. That's why those with irritable bowel syndrome (IBS) or irritable bowel disease (IBD) often experience anxiety and depression.

The gut is a good place to start if you have issues with mood regulation such as grief, sadness, depression, or anxiety.

According to Chinese medicine, the onset of grief is processed in the lung and large intestine. It's all about letting go. Overwhelmed? Constipation? Are you holding on to something? Diarrhea? Are you too anxious to even hold it for a minute?

Think about it. If *Candida* can preferentially feed itself by making us crave sugar, how are the other inhabitants of our gut driving our outward behaviour? Balance the gut, balance your life.

Think bigger. Your intuitive gut, your gut feelings, gut intuition, gut sense...where does this all come from? I know: we have a left and right side of our brain. Left for logical. Right for creative. But the gut is the intuitive. A little earlier, you met Amanda. You learned how intuitive her gut was. So much so that she felt pangs in her gut when she detected anger in her boss. We all need feminine or intuitive energy, our gut sense. Remember Maxwell?

Your solar plexus around your navel area might as well have an antenna sticking out from it. Through it, you receive information about the energies, thoughts, and feelings of people, plants, and animals around you. Its intuition brings you insights. If you are one of those extra-sensitive people, sometimes called empaths, it can be difficult to tell which emotions belong to others and which are your own. Emotional discernment and regulation are just as important as intellect.

Keep time to practice connection with your breath and regularly take time out to be quiet with yourself. As you get to know your soul, you can separate what is you, what is truth and light, and what is not.

Peel the onion.

CONCLUSION

Look how far you've come.

How are you now?

Pause for a moment and listen to any messages from your body.

What does it say?

What sensations are there?

Does it scream?

Or is there a whisper?

What through this read resonates with you most?

How have you been kind to your gut today?

MORE THAN A TUMMY ACHE

Now, does it make sense to say your gut health really does impact the health of the rest of your body? What layer of your onion are you ready to peel? Do you recognize how your life landscape contributes to the onset of your chronic health issues? It's more than a tummy ache, right? Many people do not understand how food can be such a reactive issue. Or that anger can feel like a dagger in the gut. Or that Alzheimer's or depression or any chronic inflammatory disease can be the result of gut inflammation.

Anything you take in beyond your capacity to digest at the time, be it emotional energy from the world around you, toxins, medications, food, the gut first senses, then the heart feels, then the brain thinks. It all begins in the gut, your primary sensory organ. The health of your gut is intricately intertwined with that of your immune system, nervous system, hormone regulation, thinking capacity—really, what happens in the gut knits us all together.

As you strengthen your gut microbiome and build better tools to manage and regulate your experiences in this world, you strengthen your capacity to digest your food and the world around you.

Let's go back to your intake form and the body notes from earlier chapters and see what has changed. As you learned, this is a process of evolution, not revolution; it takes time.

Make notes on areas in which you would like to improve further.

Think of challenges to change you might have.

Remember all the work you did on the gut microbiome? This

makes a big difference in your food tolerances. If you find you still react to many foods, you need to do more microbiome work. You may wish to do another month or two of the basic protocol before trying new foods. You may wish to continue abstinence as your energy shifts and you feel better maintaining your new choices.

PEEL YOUR LAYERS

Conventional medicine will soon come to the same pages you are on here. It is undeniable that the intricate nature of gut health permeates the health of the rest of the body. This is not woo-woo stuff but scientific research, although some of that woo-woo is simply science ahead of its time. That's the wisdom I've referred to. The rest may very well be just woo-woo. How do you know the difference? Time will tell. Even in medical school, we are told that a lot of what we learn, in ten years, will be obsolete. Find this scary? Doctors and scientists are human, too. Just as it's not your fault for negatively impacting your being in ways you didn't realize, the same goes for us, the medical professionals, though we're accountable for more than one person's health. Although trained professionally, we are all doing our best to provide information and advice based on what we have been taught and what we know at a given time.

Food is a large factor in how we interact with the environment. Chapter 1 helped you understand how your environment beyond your food might impact the health of your gut. Food is a connection to others and is critical to sustaining life.

To get to the root cause of what's going on with your health, first consider how you feel. When things get so off balance that the body cannot rebalance, problems arise.

Obstacles to health can result from our own misguided choices or from traumatic events beyond our control. Regardless, as introduced in chapter 2, the body speaks. Sometimes it screams. Most times it whispers. If you are quiet enough, you will learn what's going on. It can be difficult if there is too much distraction. This is when you start by peeling the onion. As you learned in chapter 1, use your timeline to record all the physical symptoms, when they started, their intensity. Journal your experience, the sensations, ideally in raw, unaltered expression—even if the words you want to use don't make logical sense; this is the way the body tries to speak. Don't get in its way. Let it out. Have a look. Let your gut sense.

There are plenty of clues to gut health, as we learned in chapters 2 and 3. Your body is not a bunch of pieces. It is a miraculous system woven and interconnected in its operation. Knit together in simple, yet complex ways.

There is no one diet that is right for everyone. Not even a diet that is best for one person's whole life. Chapter 4 helped you discover the impacts your food choice makes on your gut and your health.

I truly believe food sensitivities have to do with the health and balance of the microbiome. Your gut flora changes, and over the course of time, major aversions to food may subside. Do the gut reset, eliminate foods to which you are sensitive and reintroduce them one at a time. Then practice the daily detox habits, the sleep hygiene routine, and your gut maintenance program along with the daily diet tips from chapter 4. Do all this for at least twelve months. Once you can distinguish the foods to which you're truly sensitive from those you just needed a break, you may opt to monitor your progress and rerun some of the gut health tests you learned about in chapter 5. Then you can refine your plans for diet and lifestyle over the next few years. Loop back like this every once in a while, and in ten years, you will be amazed at who looks back at you in the mirror. Just look at how far you've come in reading these chapters. Imagine ten years. All of this will slow your aging process and lower your risk of flares, autoimmune disease, cancer, diabetes, and other chronic disease. It's all about constant improvement.

Food sensitivities can definitely make one hypervigilant and admittedly a bit obsessive. The thing is, if you know what to do to make yourself feel good, you really want to do it. Food becomes an issue of nutrition and safety first and of socialization second. The difference in how you can feel and function is definitely worth it.

There are many ways to climb the mountain. If one path doesn't work, try another. Once you've gone through the gut reset in chapter 6, you don't necessarily have to go through it again. You might like to do a mild weed or rebalance of your gut microbes once or twice a year. Depending on your genetics and environmental factors, it may be a good idea to continually take a probiotic to back up the good guys. Ongoing, it only makes sense to include some fermented food and feed your microbiome with plenty of fibres and prebiotics. Individualized medicine is key. There is no one-sized-fits-all solution. You can hack away on your own, but you'll likely be much more successful with some testing and a trained eye to guide your journey.

Generation over generation, our needs as a society will change, and so will our medicine. What I find so assuring are the tried-and-true traditional medicinals, the things that big science won't invest in because no one can patent them as their own. They are owned by our great creator. They ought to be studied and honoured. As you learned in chapter 6, they are timeless and effective.

Chapter 7 helped you gain hold of your challenges to change. Tease apart what comes first: food or mood? Remember, emotions need to be felt. Emotions are energy, too. Discern what are yours and what belongs to others. Do this and set appropriate barriers, standards, and criteria. Then as you hold space, don't ignore your emotions. Don't put them in charge either. Take what you need, learn from it, make plans where appropriate for response, and let go of the rest.

Daily routine is important. The body loves routine. Energy needs to move and flow. I include outdoor activities to get fresh air and keep me connected with nature. I like to walk and sing or say a morning prayer when I go outside each morning. Then partake in some cardio and weights, or maybe just yoga. It lets me get a hold of the day before it gets hold of me. I practice good sleep hygiene. Even at that, if I experience periods of poor sleep, I will do a lymphatic massage or castor oil packs for thirty minutes with heat to help move lymph. The appendix includes a daily detox handout and a lymphatic handout.

Chapter 8 highlighted why meal timing and hours of daily digestion make a difference in your blood sugar, gut lining, memory, mood, and cardiovascular health.

Remember, you do not live on food alone. Chapter 9 highlighted how stress affects the health of your gut and, ultimately, your immune system. Prayer, breathing, yoga, and regular exercise are critical to your health.

The importance of daily connection goes without saying. This is your lifeline. There is no way a body can heal without a little (or a lot) of Divine intervention. Call it what you wish; we are not here alone. You are not alone. Yes, we need social interaction with other fellow humans, pets, and plants, but an honest connection to your creator is so critical to your well-being.

Healing will come in layers. Yes, like an onion. Constantly peeling back. Each time you start over, you go through the physical, emotional, and cognitive layers. To keep all those healthy, you can't be rotten at the core. Your core strength will come from your connection, the premise of chapter 10. Like your gut health, your spiritual health will permeate outward to the rest of your body. Whether you do this through the breathing exercises developed by the HeartMath® program, daily devotion, prayer, walks in nature, meditation, small-group study, or all of the above, you need some way to find light in the midst of darkness. It is not about religion. It is about faith that truth will prevail and that there are bigger things in the works than those you see before your own eyes. That's trust.

Chapter 11 taught that when you trust gut senses, you honour the connection between your soul and the greater powers that be; you balance the female and male energy, your yin and yang. When you allow yourself to be in a safe place, you let down your guard, you are less anxious, you rest. Only then can you truly digest both food and the world around you. You now have tools to manage what you once felt was beyond your capacity to digest. You transform energy from your food and environment into the essence of not only who you are physically but also spiritually, as your soul.

FINAL WORDS

"What's in the parcel on the front porch?" my husband calls to me as he approaches. I respond, "It's my sample getting shipped to the lab." He responds with a big, loving smile. "Oh, so it's your shit at the door. That's all you had to say."

Guess I finally got my shit together! Over the past few of years, I have to admit, I'd never done a stool analysis. I guess I was listening to my gut sense after all. I'd been researching and learning and applying but never measuring. I'd sensed that way of doing things was effective. But now I wanted to know for sure. I have only one body, so it's best I take care of it with what I know now. Now I can balance science with wisdom. One should ultimately reflect the other.

The email with the results arrived. I have to say, I am excited and happy to report my regime is working quite well.

Hippocrates was truly wise beyond his time. The health of the gut really does make deep impacts on the health of the entire body, mind, and soul. We just needed 2,450 years of science to catch up with him! Or we could just trust our gut more.

In this book, you have learned how to:

- Get to the root cause of your health problems
- Identify clues your body gives about your health
- Create a personalized eating plan
- Become familiar with tests that can evaluate gut health
- Approach a gut reset protocol
- Deal with challenges of change
- Get better sleep (and why this is related to gut health)
- Develop skills to manage stress (and why this is related to gut health)
- Tune into your inner wisdom—build your core strength

I have also:

- Given you tools to support the detoxification process
- Illustrated how you may maintain optimum health

Peel the onion.

One layer at a time.

APPENDIX

TIMELINE

GENETIC INFLUENCE
(Family medical history or
significant genetic report data)

Notes about you/your mother
in prenatal and birth

	LIFETIME TRIGGERS AND SIGNIFICANT EVENTS
Date (Age)	

	DISEASE DIAGNOSED
Date (Age)	

Current Signs and Symptoms	

	DATE STARTED/DOSE/PURPOSE
Current Medications	

Current Supplements	

WEEKLY DIET DIARY

	Monday	Tuesday	Wednesday	Thursday	Friday	Saturday	Sunday
Breakfast							
Lunch							
Dinner							
Snacks							
Comments							

Name: _____

Start Date: _____

A BETTER WAY TO REQUEST A DIETARY RESTRICTION

As you can see from this example, keep it simple!

To: Joanne Winifred

From: Laura Brown

Date: Wednesday, November 27, 2019 4:40 p.m.

Subject: Dietary restriction for guest November 30

Hello,

I tried to call; however, you are now closed.

Wondered if it were at all possible to have help with dietary restriction as a guest with Southwestern event on Saturday, November 30.

Meal prep is:

(1) celiac disease (absolutely no gluten, which includes Worcestershire sauce, soy sauce)

(2) dairy-free

If you are not sure how to accommodate, essentially a salad with olive oil and a wedge of lemon with some grilled chicken usually is a safe bet.

Please let me know if this is possible, given the context of the event of which I am unsure.

If it is not possible to accommodate, please let me know so I can bring my own food.

Thank you so much.

Warm regards,

Laura Brown

On November 28, 2019, at 8:34 a.m., Joanne wrote:

> Hi, Laura, we will be able to accommodate your gluten-/dairy-free meal. I will forward this to our kitchen staff.
>
> Thanks, Joanne

I always say celiac because it is easier than gluten-free; it emphasizes the care I need in my meal preparation. I have to admit, I was still a little worried about food security! But it was fine. I ended up with a full meal of antipasto—melon with prosciutto, salad with oil and vinegar dressing, gluten-free pasta and sauce, roast chicken, and potatoes. Good, simple cooking with natural ingredients. Italians did it up right that night!

SLEEP HYGIENE

MINIMIZE OR AVOID STIMULANTS

- Avoid alcohol (wine, beer, and hard liquor) within three hours of bedtime.
- Avoid caffeine-containing beverages and foods after 1:00 p.m.; if sensitive to caffeine, avoid them after 10:00 a.m. (These items include many sodas, energy drinks, teas, coffees, lattes, and chocolate.)
- Reduce sugar
- Avoid foods to which you are sensitive.
- Consult your pharmacist and doctor to determine whether your medications contribute to sleep problems. Do not discontinue them without permission from your doctor.
- Complete any high-intensity aerobic exercise before 6:00 p.m. (or at least three hours before bedtime).

ROUTINES TO AID IN SLEEP

- Plan your sleep; 8½ to 9 hours in bed.
- Train your biological clock; go to sleep and wake up at the same time each day.
- Go to bed before midnight.
- Avoid late-afternoon or evening naps.
- Avoid naps longer than forty-five minutes unless you are sick or quite sleep deprived.
- Avoid large meals or spicy foods before bed.
- Finish all eating three hours prior to going to sleep. Have a small bedtime snack of protein and fat (nut butter is excellent) only if necessary.
- Avoid drinking more than 4–8 oz of fluid before going to bed.
- Take a hot salt/soda aromatherapy bath. Raising your body temperature before sleep helps induce sleep. A hot bath also relaxes muscles and reduces tension. Add 1–2 cups Epsom salts (magnesium sulfate absorbed through the skin is very relaxing) and ½ to 1 cup baking soda (sodium bicarbonate, which is alkalizing to a stressed-out, acidic body) and ten drops lavender oil (helps lower cortisol levels).
- Consider reading a good, neutral black-and-white book under low light.
- Don't stay in bed more than twenty to thirty minutes trying to fall asleep. Leave your bed and go to a relaxing room other than the bedroom and try breath focus or other meditation.
- If you awaken early because of unnatural light, wear an eye mask.
- If you awaken early because of recurrent thoughts, write them in a journal. If this does not help, consider counseling.
- If you snore or wake periodically with intense anxiety, get a sleep test done. You may have sleep apnea.

- Try a weighted blanket to feel more secure while sleeping.

BEDROOM AIR QUALITY

- Keep your bedroom air clean.
- Use HEPA air purifiers/filters.
- Use the filter on a low setting at night if the noise is soothing. Otherwise, use the filter on a medium setting throughout the day.
- Humidity in your house, especially your bedroom, is best at 45–55 percent. Hardware stores sell humidex readers. No, the humidifier on your furnace is not enough.
- Too much humidity is an issue. If you see mold or have a musty smell in your bedroom, have it checked or cultured for mold with culture plates. If there is mold, have the house evaluated for water leaks and air quality issues to be fixed and see that the mold is cleaned appropriately.
- Consider cleaning the vents in your house once a year; change your furnace filters regularly. How often you should change it depends on the type of filter.
- Avoid toxic glues and other odorous items. New furniture, plastics, vinyl flooring, and paint can all affect indoor air quality. If you have to introduce these, open a window for as long as possible.
- If your nose is blocked and you have trouble breathing through it, take the above steps and consider using a saline spray, neti pot rinse, or breathe-easy strips.
- Lymphatic pump at the clavicles may also help relieve sinus congestion. See "Lymphatic Treatment" later in this appendix.

LIGHT, NOISE, TEMPERATURE, AND ENVIRONMENTAL ISSUES

- Turn down the light in rooms you are in fifteen minutes before going to bed.
- Decrease the light in your bedroom by using a dimmer or a reading light with a dimmer.
- Use dark window shades or consider a set of eye shades or an eye mask.
- Decrease irritating noises in your space by closing windows, using earplugs, or using a white noise generator or a HEPA air filter.
- Turn off or remove any appliances or clocks that make noise.
- Make sure your sleeping area is in the correct temperature range (neither too hot nor too cold).
- Remove possible sources of electrical fields near your bed: electrical outlets, clock radios, stereos, cell phones, electric mattress covers, computers, and monitors. Consider powering your Wi-Fi off at night.
- Consider replacing your pillows with hypoallergenic pillows. Use ultrafine allergy pillow and mattress covers.
- Remove clutter from the room.

BEDDING AND PILLOWS

- Consider placing a side-sleeper pillow under your neck when sleeping on your side.
- Consider using a body pillow to hug and put between your knees to align your back and shoulders at night.
- Roll backwards at a slight angle onto a body pillow if you have hip bursitis.
- Sleep on the highest quality bed linens you can afford.

- Consider half-hour exposure to a blue or 10,000 lux bright light first thing in the morning if you are going to bed too late and want to shift to an earlier bedtime.

DAILY DETOX

Keep all detoxification organs healthy.

Liver

- Eat brassica (cabbage) vegetables daily.
- If you drink, limit yourself to a maximum of one glass of wine per day, and have some days when you don't.
- No caffeine, or if you must, limit to 200 mg maximum by noon.
- Blood glucose regulation
- Topical castor oil rub (not during your period)

Kidney

- Tea: nettle, dandelion, yarrow, linden
- Plenty of water to refresh

Gastrointestinal Tract

- Insoluble and soluble fibre
- Know your food sensitivities and/or allergies

Lungs

- Twenty minutes fresh air daily

- Cardiovascular exercise

Skin

- Fat-soluble vitamins (A, D, E, K)
- Sweat daily—exercise, infrared sauna
- Plenty of water to refresh

Emotions

- Feel, express, let go, and move on

Hormonal Balance

- Seven to eight hours uninterrupted sleep
  - Dark room, quiet, right temperature/humidity
  - Screen-free one hour before bed
- Daily exercise thirty to sixty minutes
- Botanical tinctures to retrain
- Seeds to promote balance:
  - Estrogen: flax, pumpkin
  - Progesterone: sunflower, sesame

Reduce Inflammation with Healthy Fats

- Omega-3: salmon, flax, hemp, walnuts
- Omega-9: raw olive oil, avocados, coconut oil, almonds

Dry Skin Brushing: Ten Minutes Daily, upon Rising

- Mobilizes immune system, stimulates lymph flow, improves

circulation, enhances removal of metabolic waste, reduces stress

- Using a soft, natural bristle brush, make small clockwise circular motions starting at the far end of extremities (hand or foot), doing the outside of each limb before the inside, and working your way toward the heart
- Order: right leg, left leg, right arm, left arm, back, stomach, figure eight around the breasts
- Follow with warm shower for four minutes to rinse away skin cells, then follow with one minute cold water

Rebounder (like a Small Trampoline)

- Mobilizes immune system, stimulates lymph flow, improves circulation, enhances removal of metabolic waste, reduces stress. Ten to twenty minutes a day

Deep-Breathing Techniques

- Mobilizes immune system, stimulates lymph flow, improves circulation, enhances removal of metabolic waste, reduces stress
- Connects to Spirit

Alternating Cold-Hot Showers

- Hot shower four minutes, followed by very cold shower for one to two minutes. Repeat three times. Always end on cold. Cold showers will also move lymph with the rapid breathing you do when you feel the cold, and the temperature contrast gets the circulation moving.

Castor Oil Packs

- Castor oil topical application, especially with heat, can be very helpful to move lymphatics and reduce inflammation (see more details in additional handout).

Top Seven Foods with High Antioxidants

- Green tea
- Red berries and blueberries
- Dark leafy greens
- Sweet potatoes, orange vegetables
- Beans
- Fish

Avoid plastics. Use stainless steel and glass containers such as Pyrex and reusable jars to store water, hot beverages, and food.

Fibre, Up to 35 g a Day

- Soluble: regulates blood sugar, excretes cholesterol: oatmeal, oat cereal, lentils, apples, oranges, pears, oat bran, strawberries, nuts, flaxseeds, beans, dried peas, blueberries, psyllium, cucumbers, celery, and carrots
- Insoluble: adds bulk, prevents constipation: seeds, nuts, brown rice, bulgur, zucchini, celery, broccoli, cabbage, onions, tomatoes, carrots, cucumbers, green beans, dark leafy vegetables, raisins, grapes, fruit, and root vegetables with their skins

LYMPHATIC TREATMENT
CASTOR OIL PACKS

Topical castor oil has been shown to increase circulation and promote elimination and healing of tissues and organs underneath the skin. It is particularly effective when absorbed into lymph circulation, which can improve digestion, aid the liver in detoxification, support immune function, and reduce swelling in injured joints and extremities. It has also been specifically used in cases of menstrual irregularities, uterine fibroid cysts, and ovarian cysts.

* DO NOT USE ON ABDOMEN DURING PREGNANCY OR MENSTRUATION. *

Modern research shows that castor oil produces the following effects:

- Enhances circulation to and from each cell by liquefying the material between cells
- Opens up lymphatic channels to increase lymph flow
- Increases the mobility and effectiveness of white blood cells, thus improving the immune response
- Softens adhesions and scarred/fibrotic tissue
- Increases prostaglandin levels, thereby decreasing inflammation

Castor Oil Pack Directions

Five nights on two nights off for three weeks

1. Use organic cold-pressed castor oil.

2. Use soft cotton such as an old sheet, tea towel, wool, or flannel. The piece of material may be reused four to five times, then discarded and replaced. Do not try to wash it.

3. Fold the material so that it has four layers, and cut it to be the desired size given the area you wish to treat.

4. Soak the cloth in castor oil in a small bowl for a few minutes.

5. Warm the pack by placing it on a hot-water bottle or hot pack before applying it to the body. Do not microwave the castor oil pack.

6. Apply the castor oil pack to the area to be treated. Once the pack is placed on the body, you may wish to place a protective plastic wrap barrier over the warmed pack or put the heat source in plastic to protect it. Cover with a heating pad on low, a hot-water bottle, or a grain bag heated in the microwave.

7. Leave heat on for limited time only (breasts, thirty minutes; abdomen, sixty minutes).

8. You may go to bed with the pack on, but take the heat away after the allotted time. Packs may be stored in ziplock bag or in a sealable container in the fridge.

9. Let the oil soak into the skin. The next morning, to clean off any oil residue, you may wash off the body with soap and water.

For quick-and-easy (but not as effective) treatment, have a hot shower or bath to warm the body. Rub castor oil directly onto the skin from the breast to the pubic bone. Put an old T-shirt on and go to bed. Shower it off in the morning.

ACKNOWLEDGEMENTS

Thank you to my husband, Gary, for all his support. Without it, I would not be who I am or where I am today. To all my patients who brought me their struggles and their stories: I no longer feel alone. To all the patients who gave consent to have their stories in this book: I am ever grateful to them for sharing. Thank you to God and my spiritual leaders. May I learn to trust you more. To Amberlea for her headshot photography, Austin for his organic garden bounty, and Mom and Dad, Heather and Russ, and all my friends for their love and encouragement. To Megan, Tijuana, Anne, Betty, and Dallas for listening and providing feedback. To Scribe for giving me a platform and a process so I could confidently journey across these pages.

ABOUT THE AUTHOR

DR. LAURA M. BROWN is a registered naturopathic doctor with a functional medicine approach. A HeartMath® Certified Practitioner and a level-2 Certified Gluten-Free Practitioner, she holds the designation of ADAPT Trained Practitioner from Kresser Institute, the only functional medicine and ancestral health training company. This means she is a wholistic expert who can recognize patterns, remove obstacles, and stimulate a body's natural mechanisms to repair damage and rebuild health.

Titled Miss Teen Ontario at age 16, Dr. Brown battled many health challenges of her own, ultimately prevailing through naturopathic medicine. She writes, gardens, hikes, swims, and entertains on twenty beautiful acres in the heart of Ontario, Canada. Learn more about her practice at southendguelph.ca.

CPSIA information can be obtained
at www.ICGtesting.com
Printed in the USA
LVHW032319150321
681644LV00028B/187